Are We Angels

A Nurse's True Stories

by

Jessica Patton, R.N.

WingSpan Press

Published in the United States and the United Kingdom
by WingSpan Press, Livermore, CA

The WingSpan name, logo and colophon are the trademarks of
WingSpan Publishing.

First edition 2020

Printed in the United States of America

www.wingspanpress.com

Publisher's Cataloging-in-Publication Data

Names: Patton, Jessica, author.
Title: Are we angels : a nurse's true stories / by Jessica Patton, R.N.
Description: Livermore, CA: Wingspan Press, 2020.
Identifiers: LCCN: 2020916452 | ISBN: 978-1-59594-656-0
(Hardcover) | 978-1-59594-652-2 (pbk.) | 978-1-59594-964-6 (ebook)
Subjects: LCSH Patton, Jessica. | Nursing--United States--Biography.
| BISAC BIOGRAPHY & AUTOBIOGRAPHY / Personal Memoirs |
BIOGRAPHY & AUTOBIOGRAPHY / Medical
Classification: LCC RT34 .P37 2020| DDC 610.73092/2--dc23

1 2 3 4 5 6 7 8 9 10

Dedication

This book is dedicated to my husband and sons, who are my everything and have been so patient and supportive of my work and writing. It is also dedicated to nurses everywhere, who work so hard to make a difference, and the patients and families who have to deal with the American healthcare system.

Contents

Prologue 1

1 The Child 7

2 Ronnie 14

3 The Dog 34

4 The Foot 41

5 The Gift 49

6 Michael 58

7 Daisy 63

8 The Bell 68

9 Quitting 80

10 Sleepover 83

11 The Priest 91

12 Choices 103

13 Ethan 110

14 A Not-So-Typical Work Day 128

Epilogue 134

Afterword 137

Prologue

For me, it's a daily struggle, being a nurse. There are two of me. One has high ideals and wants to make a difference. The other is tired. It takes every ounce of energy to get up on the days that I work, put on a smiling face and go. Financially, I am trapped. I need the job. My family depends on me. And, like most people, I need health insurance. I'm at the top of the pay scale, which means I'm old and expensive, basically no longer hire-able. Employers have a field of young eager nurses to choose from. I question why I ever wanted to become a nurse in the first place. I have been a nurse, now, for more than twenty-nine years.

I debated how I should begin this book, mainly because I originally sprinkled it with sugar-coating describing the miraculous discovery of my curiosity about what it would be like to be a nurse. This is what people usually see. People make comments such as, "Oh, nurses are so wonderful. They are truly angels." Hogwash! I don't mean to be blunt, but I'd like to set the record straight. It's an unspoken belief, a shared common ideology, that nurses are not human, nor do we have thoughts or feelings about what happens at our job. This is largely because of our professionalism. When people see our acts of kindness, patience, intelligence, and advocacy for their loved ones, their minds blur trying to interpret what they don't understand, and they chalk it up to words like "special" "angel" and "wonderful."

That's really nice. The sentiment is appreciated. If I have ever truly helped your family member, made a difficult situation easier, given my whole heart to your pain, finessed the system to help you, helped your loved one die comfortably, or started an IV quickly on the first stick, then that was worth it. That could all take place on one shift, by the way. But it comes at a cost. The nurse must be codependent and give up all boundaries and physical needs of the self to do it. But for the record I do care. I do want to make a difference. And rarely, every once in a while, I/we nurses do. Okay, maybe more often than that.

What I guess I want to say is that watching a nurse do his or her job is very much like watching a ballerina. You see the beautiful tutu, the graceful hand movements, the balance on the tips of toes, the long outstretched neck and upturned chin. What you don't see is the hours of practice, the near starvation, the open, bleeding sores on the feet, and the hateful, relentless, fierce competition. It's kind of like that.

When I was young, I had investigated several other careers while I waited tables at an Italian restaurant. One evening I waited on a woman who dined alone. She seemed tired. Her face was sullen. She wore blue scrubs and had a name badge that said "R.N." She must have been from the hospital down the road. I had made several attempts at conversation with her and she just smiled; clearly she wanted to be alone. I observed her against the mustard walls dotted with painted grapes in the dim light. She kept her brown curly head down. She had a glass of red wine and pasta with red sauce.

The rest was left up to my imagination, which was alive with curiosity. Why was she so sullen? Had she just seen someone die? What really happens in a hospital? I bet she had some stories to tell. What was so messy that it required scrubs?

Why does my mother say nursing is so hard? Yes, I was doomed from the start. You would have thought my mother would have warned me away, but she was encouraging. "You will always have a job," she said. And she was basically right. What she didn't prepare me for was the intense, most ego-deflating, disgusting, wonderful, terrible job I could have imagined and I have an expansive imagination. Picture Tom Cruise in *"Jerry Maguire"* jumping around, telling Cuba Gooding, Jr., in the restroom that it was the most back-wrenching, ego-deflating job and Cuba will never know the half of it, and you'll have some idea. But that was just football.

Most get into ballet school or nursing school and it is only after investing great time and money on our education and training for months, or years, do we realize what we've gotten ourselves into. We go in tough, accepting every challenge, thinking "I could be the one," one of the best, most caring, knowledgeable, helpful nurses ever. But with all of the stress, there's a turning point where we are faced with the decision to quit or go on.

I was faced with that decision about three-fourths of the way through nursing school. I felt I couldn't handle it anymore. Nursing school is like a prolonged boot camp. The instructors mess with your mind because they try to make you think differently, which really *is* necessary. But in my experience, as a student, and now precepting new nurses and mentoring students at our hospital, nursing school does not prepare nurses. There is simply too much work and too much useless information. No one prepares the nurse for the unexpected.

I remember being assigned to read one thousand pages, and write a thirty-page care plan, as well as study for two tests and do thirty hours of class and clinical, all in one week, and while working part-time. I stopped. I actually quit attending for a whole week, right in the middle of the semester. I look back at that time. Should I have quit? Maybe I wasn't smart enough. There would have been no shame. Over the years, I have wondered many times if I should have just let it all go.

During the week that I "quit," I cried, alone, for a long time, and thought there was something wrong with me. I felt a temporary sense of freedom. I partied hard with non-nursing friends. And after that week I went back. The day I went back, there was a test about the genitourinary system. I talked to God. I told him, "If I pass this test, I will stay in nursing school."

I ignored the dirty looks from the instructor, put my head down, proceeded to guess at each question, and totally faked it. Two days later, the test was returned and I looked down, dumbfounded, staring at the letter "B." Contrary to what *I* really wanted, I was left with the impression that God wanted me to be a nurse. The bastard. This and the general fear of failure was, for me, as real as wearing a thick winter coat, and became my motivating cattle prod. In the end, of the original sixty-three nursing students in our class, I was one of only sixteen who graduated.

I apologize for all this negativity. Maybe I'm depressed? Maybe I'm just whining? I've felt this way for a long time, about twenty-nine years. Maybe it's just me? I don't think so; most of my co-workers share the same feelings, complain with the same ragged look in their eyes, as I empathize with a pat on their back. Or they stop caring, the beginnings of "Nurse Ratched." I think the problem is, I feel so much for people. I give so much. I want to make a difference. *It's so easy to escape myself by hiding in the stories and problems of other people.*

One day at work, a chaplain, Sister Pam, was making her rounds during a particularly difficult shift. She asked me how I was and I thought, *Why not?* I let some of the sadness out. I let her in on the inner thoughts I had. I told her how unhappy I was. She said she understood that I was unhappy, then asked me, "Do you have *moments* of happiness?"

"Yes," I said. I did. This gave me pause. I did. I do.

This, and the bits of steam we nurses let off to each other, and alcohol, and the joking around, and the look of relief on the faces of patients, was how I coped. And writing. For me, journaling and writing about it has kept me sane. So here are some of my stories in all of their raw, painful, beautiful glory. All of the names have been changed with the exception of Ethan's story, with his and his parents' permission.

For your understanding, my career path was a little backward. I worked first for a children's hospital, then home health children's, mom and baby visits, then adult home care visits, then adult home infusion visits, then to an adult hospital. In the end, I'd like to say that it was all worth it.

1

The Child

I was new to nursing and worked at Children's Hospital. I worried. I worried every day that I went to work and on the days I was off. I was full of anxiety. Did I know what to do? Could I pass all my meds on time? What would I do if a child needed babysitting because the parents weren't there and I had the other children to care for? How do I get a baby to take nasty-tasting medication? Ah, the insecurity and stress of a new nurse! And like most new nurses I went right into the easiest job I could find right out of nursing school. Pediatric neurology/neurosurgery. Ha! What was I thinking? Thank God for my co-workers, my mentors.

The truth is I loved kids but I also wanted deeply to learn from these families. My childhood was rough. We moved every six to twelve months, things were always in a state of drama and chaos. I knew it wasn't normal. I wanted to see normal. I figured it was a fair trade: I nurtured and cared for their children in exchange for a voyeuristic observation of how the families treated each other and cared for each other and handled stress. I watched.

And it worked for the most part, and I learned and grew as a nurse and a person. There were all kinds of things to see.

Are We Angels

There was a saying, "Come on in folks, drop your kids off here at 'Hotel Children's Hospital'! We'll fix 'em up and call for pickup when they're done." Some parents would actually do this. The horrified little face that they left behind was ours to love and care for. And we did our best, and I was on the night shift, the scariest time of all for them. These were the heartbreaking cases.

One that comes to mind was a three-year-old girl, who had been in her safety seat on her mom's bicycle when her mom had an accident. The little girl was injured, her neck broken. She would be paralyzed for the rest of her life. Her mother suffered from guilt that penetrated every cell in her body. It seemed to have cost her her marriage. I often wonder if their story is one of the reasons we no longer see bikes with toddler seats above the front wheel by the handle bars, or behind the seat.

Her father visited separately, in the evenings. The wide halls with carpeted floors were dimly lit to encourage sleep. He would play on his harmonica "The Carnival Is Over," to help her relax. Its long slow notes drew out the innocence of childhood. The drops of melancholy mixed with the hopeful melody echoing in her room and out into the halls, hypnotized the children and their nurses.

Then there were the miracle kids. There were kids who had a certain type of Cerebral Palsy who walked in on tiptoes or bow-legged with crutches, who would have dorsal rhizotomy surgery. A little recovery time and physical therapy and they would walk out of the hospital almost completely normally. There were lots of tears of joy and sighs of relief from parents, who were eternally grateful to God and the M.D. (also referred to as "mighty deity"). Truly it seemed to them that there was no distinction. The miracle of the possibility of a normal life, defined as not having to work twice as hard every day at everything compared to most other people, or other children, was a reality. And it was shocking and it was beautiful, and it was real. I loved to drink those memories in, and there were many other miracles and surgeries and treatments to observe and celebrate, and children to care for and play with. And I had the best seat in the house.

But there was this one story concerning one family that haunted me for years. It caused me to secretly question everything I knew, everything I believed about life, and God and love and death and reality. I don't remember the child's name but I remember his spirit. Let's call him Timmy.

It was just another day and I was tired again. I slept before my twelve-hour night shift. I slept afterward. I never seemed to get enough sleep. The beginning of my mounting anxiety, old and reliable, was waking me up. I was thankful for its consistency. I showered and put on my jacket over my white scrub pants and pink top. I drove to work and threw my stethoscope around my neck, the one with the light grey koala bear strategically mounted on it, put on a smile, and left my troubles at the door.

I was listening to our daily tape-recorded report with the other nurses (okay, now my age is showing). He wasn't my patient but I heard about little Timmy, five years old, and his brain tumor. We gave chemotherapy at Children's. And I hated it. "Giving chemotherapy at Children's" was a phrase that shouldn't exist. Those words didn't belong together. Which was probably why the public did not see this on a daily basis. No one wanted to believe it was real. Being a nurse sometimes felt like living in a war zone. Real children were happy and healthy and playing ball and dancing and raising their hands in class. Real kids didn't have cancer. But real kids really did.

Timmy was five. He was fair-skinned with blond hair and big brown eyes. I had to peek in on him. He was beautiful. And small. I must have stared for about five seconds, then quickly moved away from the door. The vision was like a wood-burning pen carefully scorching the image into my woodblock-headed brain. I tried to resist but it was too late. It was there. A mother with bobbed brown hair and bangs was sitting with Timmy's little sleepy body curled up on her lap, a book in her hands, his homemade choo-choo-train patchwork quilt half fallen from his lap.

She was rocking him back and forth and reading a story, and in a fraction of a second, it occurred to me that it was bedtime. *We read stories at bedtime.* This mother was reading because now it was time to forget. It was their time to dream. In that moment full of kings and queens and beasts and bows and magic potions and princes and horses and rainbows, there was no cancer. There was no nausea, there was only their love and their story. *How peaceful was forgetting* I thought. *How completely full of newness and hope.*

The prognosis was grim. He would die from this. No matter how much his parents begged and pleaded and prayed and researched and screamed and wept, they could not protect him from this. The unimaginable would happen. Little Timmy, a forty-pound bundle of life and love and giggles and squeals and questions and wonder and potential and innocence would one day *not be*. How did his mother cope with this? How did she get through her days? I could barely contain my tears and he was not even my child! I didn't have children yet. He was not even my patient.

This all seemed intolerable to me. I was only an observer, yet I could imagine how helpless and powerless this mother felt. I imagined how she would open her eyes in the morning half asleep, having forgotten, and would breathe and think about her family with peace and love and things to do and deadlines, and then it would hit her. She would remember. And like a book bag, packed way too heavily with way too many books, she would feel the weight of remembering again that Timmy had cancer. And she would try to stand up but it would be too heavy. She would have to wait a minute and first summon all of her strength. Maybe she could remove one or two books, to try to numb the pain for a while. She could rise and let her body acclimate to the heavy load and begin another precious day of forced cheerfulness.

In my thoughts she would want to pray but lately had been too angry with God. In fact, she hated him. She was thinking she may stop believing in him. Because God had done worse than taken her happiness: He had taken her hope. So she had to do it all herself, now.

Back in his room the next morning, in reality, I peeked in again as she carried her virtual backpack of weight over to Timmy's hospital bed and conjured up the best smile she could, crawled in and kissed him gently. She cuddled up to him, his little body completely relaxed, his face like a cherubs', peaceful. Blissfully unaware. She folded him into her arms, trying to absorb some of his peace, to throw the books off, to sink deeply into mindlessness, forgetfulness, peace and love of this wonderful being. And she did for a minute, but then she remembered. They were being discharged today.

Timmy would go home on hospice. Another contradiction in terms, pediatric hospice. No more needle sticks, no more medicine that made him sick, no more CT scans, MRIs, PET scans, blood pressure checks, lab results, lights flashed in his eyes. No hope, only comfort. She began to cry. Then she panicked. She didn't want him to see her cry! But the dam had burst now and she carefully moved away, burying her head in the pillow. Timmy stirred and opened his sleepy eyes, saw his mommy and knew. He knew his mommy loved him and he seemed to also know that everyone had a breaking point. But somehow this child also knew it would be okay. (His mom had told us, before their discharge, about this conversation.)

"Why are you crying, Mommy?" he asked, but he already knew the answer. His mom tried to calm her breathing and form some simple words for him but was unable to, and it all came tumbling out.

"Because you're going to go to heaven, honey, and I will

never get to see you or hold you again. And I'll never get to laugh with you or kiss you. I won't know if you will be okay. I won't be able to take care of you and protect you and watch you grow." Tears streamed down her face. The heaviness from her back then rested in her gut, as if the books were now bricks. She held her abdomen with one arm and Timmy with the other.

And this beautiful, tiny, sweet, cherub-faced child with the wisdom of a monk lay there caressing his mommy's hair and said, "Don't worry, Mommy, I'll be just fine. And when I get there I will send you a rainbow to show you that I'm okay."

Somehow she stopped. She looked into her little angel's eyes, and somehow believed him. For the first time in a long time, she had peace.

"Okay," she said. She could breathe again, and they went on with their day.

It must have happened quickly because about a week later, the hospital floor was all a buzz. There had been some news. It had been raining outside, a sort of on-again off-again series of spring thunderstorms, with a familiar Midwestern tornado siren here and there.

He had passed away about four nights before, at home, in his father's arms. The day after he had passed, on the evening news was a story of the most brilliant rainbow stretching across the sky from east to west, as far as the eye could see. I had caught it out of the corner of my eye, and at the time thought it was nice, but didn't think much of it. But then I remembered the story. Her words came back to me in a rush of adrenalin. The rainbow was for her.

At the hospital, my co-workers were passing around a piece of paper. It was a poem Timmy's mother had written. It described Timmy and his family and the horror and pain, then the promise and the rainbow. It detailed the events mentioned in this story, which is how we found out and how I was able to write about it. Thirty-some years later I still have a copy of the poem.

I hope she had found some peace amidst burying her son. Did the miraculous confirmation that he was okay calm her aching heart? I can only guess that she would be able to move on. I imagine she grieves still.

I wondered what happened to her faith? Was it restored with the appearance of the rainbow? I wondered about my own children. I ached for them. I wondered how God functioned, in the light of all of this. I wondered about war and anger and brutality and human pain. I wondered why we suffer, and was not satisfied with the old story about an apple. I questioned justice. I began a lifelong study of the who, what, why, where, when and how of us. I searched for the why of love, of hate, of suffering. I searched for meaning, for truth.

I wondered, would I find peace? Would I have a happy marriage? Would I have children? How could anyone cope with the loss of a child? I wondered if it might happen to me—no, I don't want to even imagine that. None of us do.

I don't know where the answer lies. I think it's different for each person. I think the solution is as simple and complex as each human being is. I think not knowing is like having faith, and marks the beginning of your journey which is as unique as you are. For me, maybe, happiness can be found in the present moment of forgetting, in loving who I have, and have had, in my life. It brings me peace. I think Timmy would have wanted that for us.

2

Ronnie

I had left Children's Hospital. Ronnie, an older woman, was a patient when I began doing regular home care visits, which I did for a few years before working with home infusion. I was learning and taking care of adults, and we were seeing Ronnie for a wound on her heel. We, the home care nurses, saw her daily to dress her wound. Ronnie lived with her husband in a beautiful area. They employed many people as maids, groundskeepers, and of course, nurses. I was learning, too, that I was a bit green, insofar as dealing with the general public.

I had been visiting her for about a month. Her wound never seemed to heal. On this day, as I had done many times before, I drove up through the wrought-iron double gates and parked on the large rounded-cobblestone driveway. About six other cars were parked comfortably there to the side in the shade, under some aged, sturdy oak trees covered with vibrant green leaves. I entered the brick and stone villa through the tall solid walnut door with gothic iron hinges, and was welcomed by Mary, one of Ronnie's maids. She wore jeans and a t-shirt, and tennis shoes, the better to run with.

"Hi, Mary," I greeted her.

"Hello. How are you today?" she said.

"Fine, can't complain. I get to be out driving around all day seeing patients in this gorgeous weather."

"Oh, nice!" She looked behind her, then said in a hushed voice, "I'm glad you're in a good mood. Maybe it will counter Ronnie's."

"Why, what's up?"

"She fired Maggie last night," she sighed. "I saw it coming. Maggie 'sinned' and took some of the food Ronnie wanted thrown out," she said. "None of us ever last more than six months here."

"Really?"

"She's impossible," Mary said, fanning her fingers out, then resting them on her thighs. She rolled her eyes.

"That bad, huh?" I said.

"Use your imagination. Then multiply by five. I know my time is limited, too. I've been fired four times and I don't know why, but I just come back. She pays well, that's why. I think I'm the only one who's lasted a year. I may hold the record!" She laughed.

I had heard there were problems. I tried to stay out of politics and drama, though. Then something occurred to me. "I might know someone who could help if you think she's interested in a replacement."

"You do? That would be great!" she said, but warned, "It may only be for six months or so. Either your friend will quit or she'll be fired."

"It's my sister," I told her. "And I would warn her. It may work out because I'm not sure that she wants anything permanent now anyway."

Mary shook her head while considering it. "As long as she is warned that it can get really bad," she said as we walked in. I agreed.

The foyer had a light brown marble floor. The walls wore neutral beige with dark-stained baseboards and crown moldings.

A glass chandelier with a few pieces missing hung in the foyer. It opened into the great room where most of Ronnie's living was done. There she sat, perched on her soft leather couch, with clutter strewn about. The dark hardwood floor was covered with a tan shag area rug. The ceiling reached about fifteen feet above. A ledge up the side of one wall formed a hallway on the second floor that was protected by black decorative railings, and must have led to the bedrooms.

"Hi, Ronnie," I said.

"Hi," she replied. Her voice was nasal and piercing, her words strangely sloppy. She smacked her mouth when she spoke and stumbled over her words. She ended her sentences with an upward inflection as if almost asking a question. There was an informal presence about Ronnie that seemed incongruent with her surroundings. It was almost friendly. It drew me in and made me want to go out of my way to be kind, especially because the reports indicated that she was a little nutty. I wanted to gain favor, to be helpful. I wanted her to like me, maybe as insurance. I wasn't sure why. Maybe it was protection against the unknown. I felt it was a self-delusional challenge, as if somehow I held the key to bringing out the normal side of her. I was naive.

"How are you?" I asked.

"Oh, it's been problem after problem here." She was not fully present, flipping through some papers, only half conscious that I was there. She always wore polyester, with the same necklace and bracelet. Her red hair was short and curly on top, but flat on the rear left. It was not hers.

Once when I visited her a man was there with a full display of about twelve wigs lined up at attention, for her inspection. She took a long time deciding. She made me wait about twenty minutes while she picked and prodded at them. I didn't know why she wore wigs. The poor fashionably dressed man had been there a while, I saw, because of his swaying back and forth and agreeing, overly so, with every critique and comment that she made. She apologized for being difficult, but then continued to be difficult. She was always specific about thanking people for accommodating her. She ended up buying six of the wigs, a good trade off for his time, for the only traveling wig salesman I had ever seen.

She finished her paper shifting while I waited silently, then stuck out her arm. "I hope everything's okay," I offered, wrapping the blood pressure cuff around her arm and pumping it up. She knew the routine. I put the thermometer in her mouth and took her pulse, and counted her breaths, or respirations.

"I had to let Maggie go," she said through her nose, rolling her eyes.

"I'm sorry," I said, and offered no more.

"Now I'll be short for the holidays and there's so much to do."

"That's too bad," I said, gathering up my courage to ask the question.

"It's hard to find good help," she sighed.

"My sister is looking for work right now. Her name is Jill. She's very reliable," I said casually. This was probably against the rules somewhere, but I couldn't think of which rule exactly. I slid the box of supplies from the side of the couch to where she sat and pulled out a plastic trash bag.

"Really? Well, that might work. Could you have her call me?" I squirted hand cleanser on my hands, put gloves on, cut the wrap off of her old dressing and removed the gauze and packing. I poured the saline over the sterile cotton-tipped applicator (like a Q-tip) and inserted it into the wound on her heel, gently twisting to clean its inside, about two centimeters deep, then pulled it out. It was not painful for her.

I thought of the safest scenario. "I tell you what, let me talk to her. Then if she is interested, I'll give you her number. Does that sound okay?"

"That sounds good," she said with her upward inflection of voice. I could tell she was interested, but her face had no expression, as always.

"Good," I said, packing a thin strip of gauze back into the wound with the applicator. I redressed the outer wound with a gauze 4X4 and gauze wrap, then taped it in place. For a month I had come, always to do the same thing. The gauze acts as a wick to allow drainage to come to the wounds' surface, so it can heal from the inside out. Eventually, in theory, the new tissue would grow on the inside and it would no longer need to be packed. Her wound should have healed weeks before.

"Okay, I'll let you know. See you tomorrow," I said.

"Sounds good. Thank you." She said through her nose, still looking down. But she sounded hopeful.

Later that evening I spoke with my sister Jill. I gave her the information, how she would basically be doing housework and cooking and whatever Ronnie needed. I also warned her that Ronnie could be difficult and not to expect to work for her more than six months or so. She was interested and I spoke with Ronnie the next day and gave her Jill's phone number. Jill was hired for ten dollars an hour, which in the 1990s was a lot.

Jill was an instantly trustworthy person, younger than I, very warm and friendly and inspired a protective instinct in whomever she is with. Mary liked her and they worked well together. I continued to see Ronnie and treat her non-healing wound for several months. The doctor would change the wound care every so often but also wasn't sure why it wouldn't heal. The doctor ran a few more tests but nothing showed as a reason for non-healing.

I saw her about three days a week because the schedule at work varied all of the time. Other nurses visited her on the other days. I was pulling up in my car to visit again when I noticed more cars than usual in her driveway. I knocked and Mary answered.

"Hi, how are you?" she said, moving quickly inside. I followed.

"Good. Does she have company?"

"Yes. Linda and Sharon are here. They used to work for her. She invited them over for lunch," Mary explained.

"Am I going to have to wait?" I asked, not sure if this would be a quick visit or a lengthy one.

"Probably not. I'm not sure, though. She's been in rare form." Mary, now whispering, said, "They're getting a divorce. She's been all over the place. She made us make twelve homemade pot pies yesterday, then yelled at us because she then said she wanted fifteen. Then she wanted them all frozen after we rushed to make them. We threw out three barrels of pasta, too. She just bought them last month and said it's gone bad."

"Barrels?" I thought she was kidding.

"Actual barrels. She has about twenty of them in the basement. She keeps five shapes of pastas, ten different kinds of chocolate chips: semisweet, milk, peanut butter, raspberry, and more things, all in big Ziploc baggies, sealed and dated, in barrels. I had to call Straub's this morning and put an order in for more. Then, this morning she had us make five quiches for lunch today. There's only six of us here!" she moaned. "We'd better get in there."

My blood pressure cuff was pulled out before I made it to the couch.

"Hi, Ronnie," I said briskly.

"Hi, Jessica," she replied through her nose. "We're having a little informal lunch here." She motioned to her guests who were across the room. I gestured a "hi" to them.

"Smells good. Mary must be a good cook," I said.

"Would you like to join us?"

I thought for a minute. I almost felt a warm, fuzzy feeling inside. I finished her blood pressure and temperature and was on to her dressing change. It was lunchtime.

"I guess I could." The smell was intoxicating. "Thank you."

I finished her wound care and asked to use the bathroom to wash my hands properly. My sister Jill was off that day, at a doctor's appointment. Mary set another place at the table, brought in two quiches and set them out. There were juices of orange mixed with lemonade. Ronnie hobbled over to the table and sat at the head.

"This is Sharon and Linda," she said. "They used to work here. And you know Samantha and Tammy, right?"

"Yes, we've met," I said, although we had never met formally. I smiled and nodded. Mary served the quiche, which looked divine, all cheesy with the aroma of ham and flaky pie crust. It felt awkward, but inviting me was a nice gesture and I was hungry.

"Have you been a nurse long?" Tammy asked me.

"Yes, about eight years," I said. Everyone took a bite.

"Jessica is one of my favorite nurses," Ronnie said.

"Aww, thanks," I replied, but felt the need to be on guard. The room had a kind of electricity, a feeling as if at any moment a lamp could go flying across the room or something. "Are you all from St. Louis?" I asked. We began talking. We talked about the quiche as Ronnie complimented the help on how good it was. We talked about kids, and about movies and the holidays for a while. Then Mary nudged me under the table. She signaled me to look at Ronnie. I hadn't really paid attention, but when I looked, Ronnie was peering out of the corner of her eye at Tammy and then nodding off. Tammy was debating the relevance of the new *Star Wars* movie with Samantha and we had begun to take sides. Ronnie was no longer the center of conversation. So, she drifted off or was feigning falling asleep.

I was thinking she might fall face first into her barely touched quiche when Sharon said to her in a loud voice, "Ronnie, have you seen *Star Wars I*?"

"No, I haven't," Ronnie said, waking with a start. She took a second bite. I had devoured all of mine, as had the others. They continued talking, changing the conversation to the holidays in the hope of including Ronnie, but realized that Ronnie was continuing to doze off. I thought this was odd. After a few more minutes I excused myself, thanked Ronnie for lunch, and Mary walked me out.

"Why was she falling asleep?" I asked Mary.

"Because she wasn't getting all of the attention," she replied.

"I see. Great quiche, Mary, Thanks! See ya."

"Thank you. See you next time," she smiled.

"So what's with the barrels?" I asked my sister the next evening on the phone. I hadn't really heard much about how it was going with her working there. I had heard bits and pieces but we had both been busy.

"She's preparing for the year 2000." That sort of made sense to me. She was storing up in case all of the computers crashed at midnight when it turned to the year 2000 at midnight on New Years', a phenomenon termed Y2K. Other people stored things, too. Maybe not as much, but I even had some canned food and water in my basement. Just in case.

"But why prepare ahead of time to throw it all away and then do it all over?" I asked. The "millennium" was about two months away.

"Who knows? You do what Ronnie tells you to do. Did you know she has ten refrigerators in her basement?"

"No! Why?"

"To store food. And she never eats it. It is a nice benefit snagging all of the food she throws away, though. The girls have taught me how to not get caught!" she said. I laughed.

"Why does she throw it away? I mean, what a waste! Why does she make so much?"

"There's no logic at all. She tells me to clean the silver, then halfway through bugs me about why I haven't vacuumed yet.

I think she just bugs us to get attention. It's her way of making conversation."

"Oh my!"

"Did I tell you about my designated job now?"

"No, what?"

"I am the designated jewelry caretaker. She likes me, so I have to do it."

"Yeah, okay. So why is that strange?"

Jill explained, "Once a month I follow her into a closet inside of a closet, where Ronnie has a safe. She puts the code into the safe and pulls out all of her jewelry, probably about $800,000 worth! She puts it in purple velvet bags kind of like Crown Royal bags. I take it to a place to have the jewelry cleaned. She has me drive her Lincoln Town Car ten miles away to an address that's in a kind of strip mall area, but more like offices. There is no sign on the door, just an address. I knock on the opaque solid glass door. I don't enter. A tall, dark-haired man in a black suit opens the door just a little, collects the bags quickly, thanks me and closes the door."

"That's creepy!" I giggled, but realized the implications. If anything were to happen to Jill on the way there, such as a car accident, and one piece went missing—what if Jill was watched and robbed?—I had an active imagination!

"Yeah! It gives me the heebie-jeebies! Then a few days later, I have to go back and get them. If anything were to happen!"

"That's like something out of a Mafia movie," I laughed. I felt protective of her. But she was a grownup. She would have to handle it. The big sister in me was coming out. "Just be careful," I said.

"I will." I was pretty sure Jill carried mace. I never saw Ronnie wear her jewelry. Jill had said she hadn't seen her wear it either. It was really none of my business.

I felt sorry for Ronnie. I knew she was at the beginnings of a divorce. I'd heard her husband found someone else. I sympathized with her and thought that this might have been the reason for her strange behavior, to draw his attention.

The next time I visited her there was another car in the driveway. Tammy answered the door this time.

"Is she with someone?" I asked. On this day, I was busy. I hoped I wouldn't have to wait.

"It's the rabbi and his wife," Tammy said.

I would have to wait. The waiting was becoming annoying. I always phoned patients the night before to set up the appointment time. She had agreed. Unless it was an emergency, she should have honored our appointment time. I was going to have to talk to her about this.

Tammy showed me in and I sat in the kitchen, where she offered me a soda.

"Thanks. You know, I'm really busy today," I confided in Tammy. Mary was there, too. "I set a time with her, but lately she's been making me wait. I have other patients to see!" I was annoyed.

"I know. She's been in rare form. My days are numbered. I'm not sure if I can take it much more," Mary said. Then we heard loud voices in the other room. We listened, although I knew it was wrong. Ronnie was talking to her rabbi and his wife.

"I don't mean to be difficult," she said. Her words were like poisoned arrows but her voice held no emotion. "I don't want to use the word "discrimination," but the leaders do seem to be more on the man's side here."

"Oh, no!" The rabbi's voice trembled. "No, we care about what you both are going through."

"I feel like no one's been on my side and I'm thinking about talking to someone about it."

Tammy went in to rescue the rabbi and his wife. She knocked on the door to the study and told them I was waiting. The rabbi quickly took his wife by the elbow and excused himself, clearly relieved to have been interrupted. He promised to talk to the other leaders at the synagogue. I went in and did my work.

After the visit, I spoke with the doctor and updated him on the wound status. It was not healing. He ordered a wound nurse evaluation. She did her assessment a few days later and changed the wound care again. We continued to see her.

It was mid-November, the rich Midwestern crimson, pumpkin-colored, and golden leaves had been shed from their trees, and the holidays were looming. I knocked on Ronnie's door and Mary answered.

"You're still here, I see," I said to Mary. My sister was in the kitchen.

"Yes," Mary said, putting on her fake-smiling face. "I need the money. Christmas is only five weeks away. I think you'll be interested in what she's doing today."

"Hi, Jill," I said as I passed the kitchen on the right, and continued into the great room.

"Hi." Jill was not smiling.

As I moved closer to her, I noticed Ronnie was sitting on her perch on the couch with her wounded foot up on her other knee. I wondered what she was doing. There were requirements to receiving home care, one of which was that the patient be homebound, meaning it would be difficult for the patient to leave the house because of his or her medical condition. One of the criteria for daily home visits, such as Ronnie had, was that the patient for some reason couldn't be taught to do his or her own wound care, so the nurses would have to do it every day. It was the exception to have a nurse come daily, not the rule. Most patients did their own wound care and the nurses visited once or twice a week to evaluate the healing. Ronnie's daily visits were based on her being adamant about not being able to reach the bottom of her heel to do the wound care.

Ronnie didn't flinch. She didn't stop what she was doing. Her dressing was off of her heel and she was leaning over, easily seeing and reaching her wound. She had in her hand a metal tweezers, not with a flat edge, but with tips that came to a sharp point. As I watched, she was pulling a long, pink piece of slightly bloody tissue out of the hole in her heel.

"Hi, Ronnie. Um, what are you doing?"

Her face was flat except for a slight grin. "I'm debriding (a medical procedure in which dead tissue is removed, usually by a doctor, with a scalpel). I just do it every once in a while so the doctor doesn't have to do it so much."

"Only the doctor should be doing that!" I said loudly. Ronnie kept picking at it, her face flat, her slight grin unchanged.

"It's fine," she said. I felt nauseated. It had become clear to me what was going on. I began to feel like a snake charmer, cautious of my every move.

"Can I take your vitals?"

"Sure," she said, and stuck out her arm.

I thought about what to say. I was not sure how to handle the situation. This kind of thing is not taught in nursing school. It is mostly learned by chance in the school of life. I decided to stick with the facts.

"Ronnie, I thought you couldn't do your own wound care."

"Oh, I don't, really. I just felt like I could lift my foot better because my arthritis and fibromyalgia aren't bad today."

Bullshit, I thought. But this was not a game. Technically, it was Medicare fraud, and I was placed in the very difficult position of deciding what to do about it. I felt as if my eyes had been opened. Again, I stuck to the facts.

"I am going to have to tell my supervisor that you are easily reaching your foot during this visit. I will also have to tell the doctor that you're inserting a tweezers into the wound and pulling tissue out of it." I quickly packed and dressed the wound, my hands shaking. I would document all of this in her chart. "You're not a doctor, Ronnie. You are probably harming your wound by doing this. You could hit an artery or a nerve. Please don't do this."

Her expression was unchanged: a flat, eerie grin. She did not make eye contact. She busied herself with her mail.

A part of me worried. I worried about her "firing" me. Nurses can get "fired" from a case if a patient doesn't want to see them again. I had been fired, once, by a difficult patient, and it felt terrible. The supervisor did nothing, really. It happened sometimes. They are aware that it happens. Nearly every nurse I've worked with has heard at least once in his or her career that a patient no longer wants to have him or her as their nurse. Nurses work unbelievably hard and are natural helpers, so it felt awful, like a fist in the gut, to be fired. I tried to learn from the experience. Mostly what I learned was that nurses are vulnerable to that kind of thing, and rehashing the experience made me realize that I wouldn't have done anything differently. There are some people who can't be happy or pleased.

I realized that I was going to have to report my findings no matter what. I still felt nauseated. I felt insulted. Did she really think I was stupid enough to believe it was okay for her to dig at her wound? I left and called my supervisor and let her know. She wanted to decrease the visits to twice a week, but expected resistance from Ronnie. She would look into it and let me know. Then I called the doctor, Dr. Cramer.

"You know how we have been wondering why her wound won't heal?" I said to the doctor. He was busy. He saw six to eight patients per hour in his wound clinic at the hospital. He wanted a quick, easy summary with a suggestion that he could say yes or no to.

"Yes," he replied.

"I saw her today. I walked in the room and she was openly picking at it with a tweezer and pulling healthy tissue out of it."

"I thought as much," he said, annoyance in his tone. "Sounds like Munchausen's. Just send me whatever paperwork you need to do for your visits. You can do whatever the wound nurse suggests. I'll sign the orders. I don't have time for this crap. I have lives to save." That was my order. He hung up the phone.

I was her primary home-care nurse, her case manager. What the doctor meant was, that he was not going to do any further investigation or diagnosing. It was up to nursing to finish her treatment. It basically gave us free rein to write whatever orders we thought were appropriate. He would sign them merely as a matter of staying informed on her progress or lack thereof. In other words, the care fell onto my, and my supervisors' shoulders. I was at a loss. How would we treat this patient?

Munchausen's. It was not an official diagnosis, but the doctor strongly suspected it. It is very difficult to diagnose. Munchausen's Syndrome is a psychiatric disorder in which the person fakes illness to gain reassurance, sympathy or attention. The patient knows many details about the healthcare system and its processes, much more than the average person. The patients manipulate situations. For example, they will contaminate urine specimens, or insert dirt into their IV lines. They insist that their case is always the exception to the rule. The normal rules of healthcare don't apply to them. The person would typically have a history of multiple recurrent hospitalizations and dramatic improbable stories of past medical experiences.

When I first left the pediatric hospital I did pediatric home visits for a short while. I had one patient whose mother was suspected of Munchausen's by Proxy. This is a form of abuse by a caregiver, in which the caregivers create fake illnesses for the patient in order to get attention for themselves. In that case, the mother frequently messed with her four-year-old child's nasogastric tube, pulling it out and then reinserting it back down the child's nose, down the esophagus and into the stomach, among other things. The mother complained that it would just come out, although that was unlikely because the silk tape keeping it attached was very sticky. But proof is elusive.

Munchausen's can be very difficult to diagnose or prove in a court of law. (A modern-day series about this is "The Act" a true story, on Hulu.)

I had too much rage back then, after seeing children who had been abused in various ways at Children's and in pediatric home care, to be an effective pediatric nurse. I reported things that I found, but didn't trust myself not to pound the mom's face and steal the poor child. I would have been arrested and lost any effectiveness or ability to help. The Division of Family Services of Missouri was watching the case, but those agencies were overwhelmed, with very few resources. I felt helpless to do anything about what I had seen. So, I had quit pediatric home care after a few months.

I decided to consult my resources. I spoke with Jill and Mary. Mary let me know the name of Ronnie's psychiatrist. When a patient signs initial papers with home care, there is a release that allows medical staff to contact each other, and insurance companies, and so on, for information if it relates to a patient's care. I called the psychiatrist. I left her a message indicating who I was, and requesting advice on how to handle the situation with her patient. I needed help. It was the only idea I had left. I waited a few days. She didn't call back. I called the psychiatrist again with the same message. This time she called me back.

"I am not at liberty to discuss any of Ronnie's case with you."

"But she's picking at her foot wound and despite our instructions to stop, she keeps doing it. I called you for advice on how to help her through this so we can heal her medically and discharge her. We have to be frugal with Medicare visits. Ronnie signed a release initially with home care so that we would be able to discuss her case with anyone involved in her care."

"I am not at liberty to discuss Ronnie's case with you." Click. I was at a dead end. I wondered if Ronnie paid her beyond her fees just to keep quiet. I was not familiar with the legalities of psychiatry.

"I've seen her picking at it several times now," Jill said, looking nauseated. "I think I've had just about enough, too. I think I'll stay through Thanksgiving, but not through Christmas or Hanukah. Her behavior was amusing at first. Now I feel irritated whenever I come in. I never know what she will change her mind about next and it is always about her and how we need to accommodate her. You can't expect her to be nice. If you do, she will burn you."

My supervisor lost the battle with Ronnie, who insisted she have nurses come out daily to dress her wound because, as she discussed with me, she had had a fluke day when she felt good and insisted that usually she was aching all over, especially her hips. She insisted she could not do her own wound care. Our hands were tied. I continued to see her several times a week. She seemed triumphant. I found myself no longer worrying about her firing me. I had almost hoped she would. I tried to put things into perspective, though. At least she was only hurting herself.

I arrived at her house the day before Thanksgiving. I planned to make it brief. I knew it would be stressful for her to begin the holidays without her husband, because I had heard they wouldn't be celebrating together. Ronnie had company: her two daughters, son, son-in-law and fifteen-month-old granddaughter. They were having their Thanksgiving together on the day before the holiday. I was worried that I would have to wait again.

"Hi, Jessica, come on in." Ronnie was unusually cheerful that day. She even introduced me to her family as I began her care.

"This is my son Aaron and my son-in-law Mitch," she said. I nodded hello.

"And this is my daughter Elana and my granddaughter

Cynthia, and (indicating a woman sitting across the room) that is my youngest daughter Leah." Leah wore leather pants, a t-shirt, had blue hair and a chain from her ear to her nose.

"Jessica is my favorite nurse," Ronnie said. My stomach clenched but I had to play along.

"Thank you. Hello," I said, continuing my work. Her daughter Elana was very beautiful, with dark, straight hair and a smooth dark dress and pearls. The little girl had her mother's hair, big brown eyes, wide smiling cheeks and wore a pink dress. She was very interested in my activity, and nursing bag.

"Hi," I said, smiling at her. She was very focused, so I let her have one of my gloves.

"Do you want me to change the dressing in the other room?" I asked Ronnie. I didn't feel it was appropriate in front of her family.

"Oh, you can just change it here," she said through her nose, her face flat except for the grin. Again, I cringed.

"Mom, the turkey smells good. Mary is outdoing herself, I'm sure," Elana said. There was a formality, a stiffness about Elana. She was anxious. She wouldn't sit down and relax. I tried to hide Ronnie's foot with my body while I removed the old dressing.

"Oh, yeah," Ronnie said, smacking her lips. "Mary has been working all morning." I wanted to finish and leave. I felt uncomfortable. The tension in the room was thick. The feeling was artificial. "Ouch!" Ronnie said as I packed her wound, and she twitched her leg. She had never complained of pain before, not once. I let it go and kept working.

"Sorry," I played along.

"That's okay," she said. "It's not so bad anymore." I hoped she would hold still so I could finish. Cynthia, concerned about the exclamation, had come over and stood by Ronnie against the couch to make sure Ronnie was okay. I finished wrapping Ronnie's foot with the gauze and cut the excess off, taping it in place.

I sat back and was repacking my bag and returning the items to her box of supplies when Elena suddenly screamed, "MOM!" We turned our heads to her. She came over and swept Cynthia up into her arms and stuck a finger into her mouth, pulling out a small pill. She made Cynthia open her hands and retrieved a second one. Elena looked down at the shag carpet in front of Ronnie. With her high-heeled pump, she kicked the toe of her shoe into the carpet. "There are pills all over in your carpet!" she almost whined. I looked down. I hadn't noticed. I counted seven pills just from my kneeling viewpoint.

Elena acted as if she wanted to say so much more, but she didn't. What she did say was, "We will do this in the front room!" She stormed off into the front room, the little pink-dressed child oblivious, resting on her hip, her arms slightly bent in a resting "W" shaped position, as she and her mom disappeared from sight.

Nausea caused my stomach to sink again. Ronnie's face was still affectless; only the slight grin had returned. I expected Ronnie to be alarmed, to apologize. No one said anything. Aaron, Mitch and Leah walked casually into the front room, their faces down, Ronnie hobbling behind.

"Good bye. Happy Thanksgiving," Ronnie said.

"Happy Thanksgiving." I walked toward the side door. I was in shock.

On my way out I stopped in the kitchen. Jill was cooking frantically. Mary stopped, which was Jill's cue to stop what she was doing. My jaw had dropped. They could tell something happened.

"What happened?" Jill asked.

"Ronnie's daughter had to pick up Cynthia and take pills out of her mouth and hand because there were pills all embedded in the shag carpet." I said.

Jill's eyes widened. Mary only shook her head. Jill looked at Mary.

"Leah was born prematurely," Mary said. "And Ronnie's son Aaron, he isn't quite right. You know Ronnie took all kinds of prescription medication when she was pregnant, didn't you?"

"No!" I said, horrified.

"She would go to one doctor for one drug, then another for a different drug, and on and on. Then she would go to four different pharmacies to get them filled so they wouldn't know. And of course she didn't tell any of them that she was pregnant at the time."

I didn't want to believe it was true. Ronnie had abused her children. Mary had seen a lot. She had worked for Ronnie four or five times in the twenty-five years or so since the kids were little. My eyes were truly opened. The house looked different to me. I didn't want to know any more.

"My God!" Jill sympathized. "Those poor kids." I agreed. Then I felt it.

My stomach was on fire with rage. It swelled up through my torso to my arms, neck and head until it engulfed me. Why was she like this? Was she abused as a child? Was she born this way? It occurred to me that I had never seen empathy or remorse from Ronnie. I tried to be rational. She was ill. But the rage wouldn't let up.

"God knows how those kids survived," Mary said, a distant look in her eyes. Jill and I shook our heads.

"I have to go," I said. We said our goodbyes. "I'll call you later, Jill."

I drove down the street to what looked like a quiet parking lot. I pulled in. I rested my forehead on the steering wheel. Rage consumed me. I no longer felt compassion for Ronnie. I thought of little Elena, Leah, and Aaron running around her house. I thought of what I had seen with my pediatric Munchausen's case. I saw her as a monster who tortured and used her kids to get attention. I wondered how they had survived. How did they cope? Did they ever speak up when they were actually ill, or did they never tell her, suffering in silence because they feared over-exaggerated treatment? What had they been forced to endure? What of their sense of self and self-regulation was left? What of their sense of self was surrendered to their mother's selfish ego? What fears grew while their tiny minds were neglected? Were the authorities ever involved?

I was full of hate. I could no longer take care of her. I had lost my compassion and objectivity. I let hot tears run down my cheeks and jaw. I ugly cried. I had such a clear vision that I wanted to remove my whole mind. I tried to detach from my sympathy for them but it took a while. I couldn't unsee what I had seen or un-know what I now knew. What could be done? Call the police? No, it was not new. It was new only to me.

I wondered why mental health care was so ineffective and inaccessible in our country. The suffering of the mind leaves children without roadmaps, without trust in themselves, without judgment or ability to express themselves. They are left to endure without any hope that anyone will help them. Little minds become locked inside, unable to speak of the horrors until they are older and have forgotten the details. And then there were the little bodies. I wanted no more of this.

I told my supervisor that I didn't want to go back there anymore. I told her the story. A nurse can fire a patient, too. She agreed. My sister quit, too.

They were not children but tools to her. I have since let it go as one of the many things in this world that I can't stomach, such as human trafficking or child molesters. I had to let it go. I hoped we could all forgive Ronnie, because she and all of the other really mentally sick people out there don't realize how they're hurting people. I wish mental health care was more effective and accessible. A part of me wants never to forget. Her kids were people, with hopes and dreams, and so many barriers in front of them. I hoped they kept their dreams alive. I hoped they found their voices.

3

The Dog

So it seems that growing up in America, there is a sort of subliminal message underlying simple, happy living that whispers: "You must not be content. You must want more, be ambitious, you must do it all, and you must hurry." Sometimes it suits the situation. But sometimes I forget to ignore this, and tend to be distractible, so if I'm not focusing on ignoring this voice, it creeps in so that inside I think, *Okay, I'll do more, move faster, work harder.*

Rushing was encouraged as if it were a virtue when I was growing up. And isn't it our cross to bear, the pressure that some of us accept? We take on too much. I think nurses in particular do this. We want to help people. We are helpers. But everyone else comes before us. And if there's not enough time, we skip the time meant for us. It's how we budget. We do it all, especially working parents with families, and especially single mothers and fathers. We cope with this intense stress by drinking, smoking, running, shopping, crying, yelling, eating, and the list never ends. We want to escape, then feel guilty, then over the years an apathy grows and some will stop caring. But is the busyness misguided? Some people work well in constant action and interaction. Not me. I need to slow down and process. Life can seem to go faster and faster, like an accelerating spinning top, until I can't see.

I had seven patients scheduled that day. I had started working with home infusion. It was spring and the air was cool and sweet. But I had no time to enjoy it. I had started early, about 7:15 a.m., with patients to see at 8:00, 9:00, 10:00 and 11:00 for scheduled labs, and would be zigzagging all around the city, as none of the times coordinated with the locations. I then had a 1:00 p.m. new-admission patient who would take two to three hours, and two others to squeeze in as time allowed. My goal was to pick up my two-year-old son, Connor from his babysitter, Miss LaDonna, who lived just south of the city, at a reasonable time, at least by 5:00 p.m. My husband was working forty miles away and would be late, so it was my job to pick Connor up. I had to stop by two different labs at some point as well, one of which closed at 4:00 p.m., to drop off the blood I would draw.

I kept all of my relevant patient information, addresses, tasks and so on, in a spiral notebook because it's impossible, and not recommended, to keep the laptop open while driving in the car. I was making good time that day. The early patients were finished on time, and I was able to squeeze in one more visit plus a lab drop in before seeing my new patient. The clock was ticking.

The admission was to teach a middle-aged man how to do IV Vancomycin antibiotics through a PICC (peripherally inserted central catheter, a long IV inserted in the bend of the arm that goes into a vein up to just above the heart). I also had to ask the patient about eighty questions, standard for newly admitted patients, but I had it down to a science. Still, it seemed to take forever, probably partly because I didn't stop to have lunch (and really had to pee!). If I had broken stride because the patient needed time to concentrate on learning, it could set me back a disastrous hour. At least that's how I interpreted it. So my stomach groaned and I crossed my legs.

I requested to use the bathroom before I left and to my relief, the patient was accommodating. It was 3:30 p.m. and traffic was thickening with the release of all the kids from school. Someday that would be my Connor. I thought about him all day.

I had to drive seven city miles, with stoplights every three or four blocks or so, way up to the north side of the city for my last patient, then back to the other lab down south. None of my computer work was done, but that was typical and didn't matter now; I could spend another two hours on my couch to finish it when I got home. As I drove I choked down a nutrition bar and some warm bottled water.

When I arrived to do a simple routine central line dressing change, the patient was asleep on the couch. He was about twenty-two years old. The house was old brick with older wood door jambs, baseboards and crown moldings. The furniture was old, broken and dirty. The couch sagged and the carpet was flat from wear. Cigarette smoke hung in the air from someone in the other room.

I was glad that the patient was present and hadn't forgotten I was to visit. As I walked in, I noticed light golden-colored fur in the next room. I squeezed some hand cleanser gel onto my hands and rubbed. I went on about my work of taking his blood pressure, temperature and pulse.

"How are you feeling?" I asked.

"Fine," he replied, his face flat.

"Can I see your leg?" I asked. He had cellulitis, an infection of the deeper layers of skin that causes redness, pain and swelling. He pulled up the left leg of his jeans to reveal his ankle and calf. I observed and there was no more redness. The antibiotics were working. "Looks good," I said. "You have two more doses of your antibiotic, then you can be finished. I think we have you on the schedule to take your PICC line out Friday.

It doesn't hurt to take it out at all. You won't even feel it. I need to change the dressing on it now, though, okay?"

"Okay," he said. He sat limp on the couch and held out his arm.

With clean gloves, I opened the sterile dressing change kit and put on the yellow mask. I loosened the plastic-like sticky transparent dressing from his skin with alcohol, and removed it. Next, I removed the wing-tipped blue "butterfly" attached to the PICC tube from the white Statlock stabilizing clamp, and with alcohol removed the Statlock from his skin. I put on the sterile gloves one at a time, careful not to touch anything except what was in the kit.

I removed a chlorhexadine prep sponge from the kit, squeezed to get some cleanser onto the sponge and cleansed the site where the PICC entered the skin and the skin all around it. I removed a new Statlock from the kit, removed the backing and stuck it to his skin below the PICC entry site. The blue butterfly part of the PICC line was placed into the Statlock, the two prongs fit through the two holes on the butterfly, and I snapped it in place. I took the clear dressing, removed the backing and stuck it over the whole area: the PICC entry site, and the butterfly in the Statlock. The single PICC tube with extension came out about six inches past the dressing so the patient could reach it to give himself his medication. At the end was an anti-reflux cap. I primed a new extension and cap with saline, removed the old one from the PICC tube, cleaned the open end with alcohol and put the new extension tube with cap on. I signed and dated the dressing.

"Do you have any questions?"

"No," he replied.

"Okay, maybe I'll see you then. I'm not sure who will be out to see you. They will give you a call."

"Okay, good bye."

"Good bye."

I stood up and looked again in the direction of the fur. A dog, probably a lab-pit bull mix, was turning himself around in a six-by-six-foot area in the next room, where he was "gated" in by boxes and furniture. His head hung low and his tail was between his legs. His submissive brown eyes met mine. I felt a cold puff of air on my skin while I held his gaze. At first I thought he was old but as I studied for a moment, I noticed he was young. And thin. Very thin. His ribs were visible and his stomach was sucked into itself. He looked like a doggie version of a P.O.W. A virtual red flag stood up in my gut.

I made a mental note of this as I went on. "*I need to call animal rescue about that,*" I thought to myself. In the nursing profession, it is emphasized that we are patient advocates. It is our responsibility to report abuse or suspected abuse that we witness to our supervisors and, if needed, the proper authority. This only applies to the elderly and children, though. With adults, it can be reported to a supervisor but not the police unless the victim agrees to have the abuse reported. There were no rules with regard to animals, but in my opinion, in home care, it could be implied. It was also the moral, humane thing to do.

Tick tock. It was now 4:15. I had to make it to the last lab and then to the babysitter by 5:00. It seemed I hit every stoplight on the way. "*Rattin' frattin' lights!*" I thought. I was exhausted, hungry, missed my family and had to pee again. I had two or more hours of work ahead of me still, and all I wanted was to cuddle my son and relax with my husband over a big dinner, that included chocolate. I made it to the lab at 4:45 and arrived at Miss LaDonna's house by 5:00. "*Mission accomplished!*" I thought, as she smiled and reported a good day. I scooped Connor up in my arms. The great thing about toddlers is that they can return hugs.

I didn't finish my computer work that night, which was common in our line of work. We had three days to do it. I was exhausted. The days were not all quite as busy as that one. The not-so-busy days were spent catching up. I cuddled with Connor and we played speed patty-cake, a favorite of his expressed by the rapid-fire belly giggles that came out of him. I made a sausage and rice dinner and began decompression. I made a consciously intentional effort to ignore the computer work. I figured ten hours was enough for that day, especially because I still needed to get the next day's assignments and phone all of the patients. My husband Terry had put in about ten hours as well and was ready for some Connor time, too. The days went on, then the week. Months went by.

One day as I was driving, I saw a man walking a yellow lab-type dog. I thought of the emaciated dog in the patient's house. I had completely forgotten. It had been a long time since the visit. "*I forgot to call!*" I thought. "*No, problem, I'll look up the information.*" But I didn't even remember the patient's name. I saw him only once. I had just shredded my notebook with all of the information in it because it was full and I had started a new one. I called the office but no one remembered who he was. We had him on service only a week or so, but that had been months ago!

On my time sheets, there were only random names going back about two months. I was assigned the territory of the whole city. I worked all over town. I knew he lived on the north side but had no idea what the street name was. I racked my brain. I gnawed on the inside of my cheek. I looked and looked, but couldn't even remember how long it had been. I found nothing. I even entertained the idea of going door to door in the area, but there would have been hundreds of doors. Brick houses in St. Louis were very common.

Guilt set in. In my mind I saw the dog's sagging face. I asked several of the other nurses who might have seen him. Nothing. I imagined the dog being beaten and starved by a cruel captor. I imagined that I was sent there, that it was meant to be that I had seen him. From his emaciated state I imagined that I was probably his last hope. Because I did nothing, he probably died.

Are We Angels

I could not forget those hopeless brown eyes. Hopeless, because of me. The self-loathing began. What kind of person was I? How could I have let this go by? I was rushing. That's how. I saw but didn't stop. I didn't stop. And then I forgot.

But how did one obtain absolution? I went home and hugged my dogs. I prayed for that dog. I apologized to him because I believed every living being had a spirit. I prayed for forgiveness but I was a perfectionist, and I had failed. Not the type of failure where a patient's note was forgotten in a chart, or blood was dropped off to the wrong lab. Failure that probably cost a life. I could have done something about it. They say that all evil needs to flourish is for good men to stand by and do nothing. Well, I allowed it. I did nothing. I will never forget. I made a promise never again to rush by while seeing suffering and do nothing.

I now contribute regularly to The Stray Rescue of St Louis. They receive calls about neglected and abused animals in St. Louis and rescue them right off of their tangled chains in the oppressive heat or bitter cold, or wherever they find them. They are wonderful. I lost my hero card that day. I am thankful that there are others.

I struggled with self-punishment over things like this and held on to the belief that I am just not good enough. Years later I learned that self-loathing and punishment are futile. Nurses tend to play the martyr role well, and take on the weight of the world. Becoming stuck in this mindset did nothing for me, or anyone around me. It did not make me a better nurse or person. It kept me from allowing myself to be human and make mistakes. Only by forgiving and loving myself am I truly able to pour that love out to others. And only by forgiving others their mistakes can I truly love them as well. I do listen to my gut more now, and when a red flag pops up, I stop. The world stops. Then I act right away. I guess stopping is sometimes the only way to move on.

4

The Foot

I wanted to know if the black foot rumor was true. We sat in the meeting at the home infusion office, a long table with about twelve mouthy nurses around it, munching our lunches quickly, because we needed to get back out into the field to see patients so we could end our day before the next one started. We all had complaints but tried to swallow them, because complaining or even offering suggestions never did any good. It would come out as factual accounts of problems, and then everybody would roll their eyes and the next problem would be described. Finding solutions was a thing of the past.

"I was on call last night and had two admissions and then Mr. Weber called and said he had a fever (and needed blood cultures drawn). Well, guess who was in St. Charles trying to finish teaching TPN administration (total parenteral nutrition-IV: nutrition for patients who couldn't take food and drink orally) to an eighty-year-old woman who was scared to death at having to learn to draw up and inject the vitamins and insulin into the TPN bag. Yeah, me! And I only had one set of blood culture bottles in my trunk! (Two were needed.) I had to use my other sets up on two patients yesterday and didn't have time to go back to the office to get more. I was like, damn! Call the nurse! Oh, yeah, I *am* the nurse!" Celeste said, laughing, banging her head down on the table, raising her hand as if it were a white flag. We laughed, but I knew, as we all did, what it was like; *that I had promises to keep, and miles to go before I sleep.* She had been out the night before until one-thirty, and back to work a full day this next morning.

"I had to drive all the way back to the office for more tubes and call the doctor on the way, and he was in no mood to be disturbed. Really? He gives orders. From his couch, at home. I drove from North County here all the way south to Arnold, got two more calls from patients that I trouble-shooted, while drawing the blood cultures and comforting a guy who might end up admitted to the hospital anyway! Not to mention the eight hours of computer work I still have to do-when? On my day off again? I'm so spent!"

We all were. It seemed never to end. We could never catch up.

"But I still have four more patients to see today, so let's get a move on, ladies." We all wanted to get a move on.

"That's a bad on-call night," Carrie said to Celeste sympathetically, and we all agreed.

On-call was kind of a joke. The nurse was scheduled to start at noon, but most started earlier, to see the regularly scheduled patients for the day. Then the on-call nurse would do all the troubleshooting and admitting patients that would be returning home from their hospitalizations in the evenings. All over town. There could be two admissions, even three, which involved asking eighty questions of the patient, obtaining a complete medication list, evaluating the home for safety, doing a physical assessment, writing a nursing care plan, and then, often at 11 p.m., teaching the exhausted patient how to do their own IV administration of their medication. Pharmacy might not deliver the medication to the home on time, so the teaching could be delayed, and we would be stuck at the patient's house, wasting precious time. And that didn't even include the fifty to seventy pages of computer work still left to be done at a later time. All with a Barbie Doll smile, and lots of encouragement for a frightened patient. The admissions might be fifty miles apart. In the snow. It didn't matter. The nurse would be allowed to stop only if the car broke down.

At monthly meetings we were lectured on budget cuts, and why the pharmacy was having trouble delivering medications and pumps on time, and can we do *one more task* to help them meet their computer requirements? I was surly. Okay, crabby. Sure, why not? Why should this meeting be any different? *Pile it on, boss*. It wasn't like that when I'd started working there. It had run more smoothly.

What had happened was that about every two to three months we were given a new task or responsibility, usually followed by losing one precious resource. Over time there seemed to be a point where a critical mass shifted and the workload was suddenly very heavy and over time became chronically overwhelming. It was as if your boss had you take on half of your partners clients then all of them; or simultaneously run the counter, the drive-through, and the fry station at McDonald's; or being told you would be working an extra twenty to thirty hours each week, every week. I remember several Christmas mornings opening presents with my boys, making breakfast and then having to do computer work. Because it had to be done. And those in charge were in perpetual denial of the changes. We complained and our voices fell on deaf ears. There were some trust issues.

I wanted to get going, to be out of there and on the road where I felt free, even if it was an illusion. After the meeting, Randy gave me a little report on her patients in Illinois because I was covering for her while she went on vacation the next week. Her patients were usually, well, interesting. "You know that pet rabbit Mr. Keller got from his family a few months ago?"

"Yeah." This could go anywhere. Mr. Keller couldn't eat and was also on TPN. Strangely, he watched the Food Network all day long. I had seen him before.

"His family ate it."

"No!" The realities never ceased to amaze me.

"I think they sold the cage, too." I mean, I eat meat, but—.

"Okay, tell me about your patients." I laughed, shaking my head. I needed to get moving.

We were in St. Louis, a border city on the Mississippi River. A short trek across the river and one entered another world without social climbing and power suits. The people seemed more simple, down to earth, and friendly in Illinois. There was a big Air Force base there and the surrounding small towns were populated by military families and their offspring known as "military brats."

This is all just beyond the "East Side", a small strip of land east of the river that I'm sure in its time was a booming, thriving place of middle-class living, with steel mills and barge traffic. Now it was a wasteland of broken dreams and unkempt houses. The schools scored the lowest possible rating. There was a high crime rate. The highways were illuminated with brightly-lit pink buildings and billboards advertising the finest strip clubs.

Most people avoided going to the East Side. Unless, of course, the St. Louis bars were closed. They closed at 1:00 a.m. The brave and persistent partiers leaped across the river to the carnival of pleasures, where the clubs were open until 5:00 a.m. or even later. There were numerous drugs to choose from. The all-night clubs satisfied both the dubstep lover and heavy-metal enthusiast alike.

Partiers felt welcome on the East Side. The clubs were happy to let them in and take their money and get them more wasted but would not hesitate to kick a guy out, or rearrange his face if he caused trouble. The clubs did their own policing.

It was necessary. And there were lots of nooks and crannies around the parking lots away from safety, away from witnesses.

These places that the law couldn't quite see were very much like third-world countries, right here in the middle of America, everywhere really, but invisible. The poverty can be so bad that I almost suspect there are cases of leprosy. Things are not taken care of. There is neglect, ignorance, depression, anger, apathy, violence. Cancer goes untreated and leaves huge holes in chests and solidified breasts. My father once said, "Don't act so low-class by not taking care of things." That stuck in my head. Take care of things. To let them go is to give up on life, to be "low-class." I don't remember what I had done to deserve such a statement, and it didn't upset me as much as it woke me up. God forbid I be "low class." I try to not be as judgmental as he. I also try and take good care of things.

The next week I headed over the river. I was going to see the twenty-seven-year-old woman with the black foot. We were giving her IV antibiotics for severe gangrene. I wasn't sure why but she was not a candidate for amputation. Maybe she didn't have insurance, or maybe it's because Illinois Medicaid went broke and stopped paying its bills in 2009.

Whatever the reason, there she was, in this third world country called East St. Louis. The town was a flat mathematical paper grid of perfectly square crisscrossed streets, with a few rectangles. It was a warm summer day, the oak trees with broken limbs still reaching out with their bright green leaves. I followed the road dotted with potholes over the train tracks, passing people walking on the side of the street. Birds perched on trees with outstretched wings and played in puddles on the side of the road. It always amazed me how birds could be contented anywhere. They couldn't smell poverty or see depression or feel apathy. If I were a bird I would live by a lake. Yet they lived here. Maybe they thought they could help.

I parked and locked my car. I knocked on the door. An older woman opened it. "Hi," I said. She nodded and walked into the house, motioning me into where my patient was. I tiptoed into this approximately eight-hundred-square-foot two-bedroom subsidized duplex apartment. There was very little furniture, white walls, tan carpet, lots of dirt and a huge flat-screen TV. I was there to change the central line IV dressing and draw blood. And to look at her foot. The older woman disappeared into the other room.

"Hi," I said once more, with a smile, to my patient.

"Hey," she said. And it was true. Yes, she had a black foot. I don't mean the skin was dark. I mean the foot was completely devoid of life. It looked like a piece of wood that had burned through and only the carbon shell remained. It started at the ankle and was the entirety of her foot.

The strange thing was, she didn't seem to care. Not a "trying to cover up any emotion" type thing. She seemed to *not care*. I pulled out my metaphorical poker-face mask and slipped it on. She seemed to have coped. She had painted the toenails! Hot pink with yellow stripes and a sparkly rhinestone on each nail. This was my first time seeing her, so it was new to me. I made some psychological adjustments. Maybe she had grown accustomed to it. Maybe she felt as if she still had her foot; why not make the best of it? I am reminded of when a mother holds her stillborn baby in her arms for a long time. I'm not sure what I'd do.

She lay there in her bed in the living room with her mother cooking in the kitchen. Her mother came in with a mixing-bowl full of chicken she was eating with her fingers. She didn't offer her daughter any.

"I'm Jessica. Is it okay if I get started?" The patient nodded yes and stared at the T.V. I took her blood pressure, pulse and temperature. I squirted on some hand cleanser.

"How are you? Does your foot hurt?"

"Fine, it's fine," she replied. I cleaned her PICC line tip with alcohol, attached a saline syringe, flushed, sucked back to remove waste blood, attached the adapter, popped on each tube, a green one, then a purple one, and let them fill with blood, then flushed the PICC again with two saline flushes.

"Have you remembered to clean the tip each time you give your Vancomycin doses?" To clarify, in home infusion, all patients were taught how to do their own IV medication administration.

"Yes," she replied.

"It looks clean." I donned a sterile mask, then removed the clear tape-like dressing from the PICC site and then put on the sterile gloves. The site was cleaned, dressing reapplied and then the cap changed. The tubes were labeled and bagged and the lab requisition form filled out. She stared at the T.V. I could see attempts at conversation were futile. I wasn't to be trusted; I was a stranger to her.

There was almost never any speaking around homes like this. This always struck me. The strange thing is, I am very quiet. I don't like to ramble on aimlessly about nothing. I don't feel the need to fill the air with chatter. I love to be amidst my own thoughts and have a vibrant inner life. So, the quiet doesn't really bother me. We had that in common.

I do, however, believe in manners and sharing and making connections and doing some talking, especially in the presence of strangers. None of that there. They simply didn't talk. I was an unknown to them, probably rumbling with fears and superstitions.

"Can I do anything else for you?" I stammered, packing my bag.

"No, I'm fine," she said.

As I bade farewell, I felt forever changed just a little. I heard that the pinkie toe broke off a few days later. I thought about stubbing my pinkie toe and about how I have no problems. I thought for a while. I thought that here, in the middle of the U.S., in the breadbasket of America, the Heartland of the wealthiest and most powerful nation in the world, there lived a girl with a black foot.

5

The Gift

I could have been fired for it at the time, but one time a patient gave me a really nice gift.

The way it worked in my days of home infusion: We received our assignments for the next day some time after 6:00 p.m. We were supposed to phone patients then, and give them approximate times when we would arrive the next day.

So after working all day we went home, had our laptops communicate with the server, and if there were new patients, looked up all the patient information and organized the day first by timed visits, such as blood levels of drugs to be drawn, then by location. Then, we would phone each patient. I hoped the phone number in the computer was correct and the patient wasn't in the mood for a long chat, because by that point I was pushing eleven to twelve hours into the day of a five-day workweek which included weekends, holidays and on-call time. On my days off I caught up on computer work. We were all constantly behind. If it was a good day, there would be no more computer work left to do and I could have my evening with my kids and husband after 7:00 p.m. or so.

In St. Louis, the city itself is rather small and is surrounded by many small townships in St. Louis County, whose residents made up the largest population in the metro area. I was a master at knowing these. I loved maps, and knew every zip code. I sort of prided myself on this! Okay, I am kind of a nerd.

In St. Louis, at least in my generation's time, there was an unbelievably common, frequently-asked question that every native asked other natives: "Where did you go to high school?" Let me explain. At a party or club, or social gathering, you may meet someone and enjoy his or her company. Something about you made them curious, so instead of having more conversation and getting to know you, the person asks that question. God help you if you're from out of town, because this would make the native feel nervous and helpless because he cannot categorize you. If you were from St. Louis and he learned what high school you went to, the native felt secure. He could now judge, I mean *categorize* you.

If you went to Vianney, for example, your school was private, Catholic, all-boys, exclusive and discriminating. Webster was a public school, so your parents were either artistic or blue-collar, and the kids were a bit rough but they were the best football rival the Kirkwood neighbors had ever known. McCleur was a public school with tough kids, a bit rougher. Fox was public, with the best drugs in the Midwest.

And the list went on. A native seemed forever bound by the choices his parents had made. For all of you natives reading this book, I attended Lutheran South for the first two years of high school, then moved east to the state of Maryland for the last two years of high school (they don't ask that question up there).

So I too was guilty of this mentality up to a point, and of course, my visits to people's homes gave me a first-hand look at all the towns and their people, and what they were like, and of course their houses. But instead of high schools, for me, identity went by zip codes. I thought they were, well, fun. I knew every zip code in the metro area. In the stressed crabbiness of my days then, the unusual mundane details kept me going, just as my nail polish color gave me little jumps of joy on the inside when I worked in the hospital. It's the little things.

I saw the filthiest of homes and the Taj Mahals, and this one was in Clayton, 63105. Like a little city all by itself, Clayton is the real business district of St Louis. And this was a miniature Taj and I went there because, you know, very wealthy people get sick, too.

I must confess I think one of the reasons I actually worked in home infusion for so long is because I loved seeing people's homes and how they lived. My husband had a hardwood flooring business and I ran it for a number of years while we had babies and I worked one or two days a month for home infusion to keep my hand in. We loved houses and rehabbing. We had built a house and rehabbed one at this point and it kind of satisfied my alter ego to visit people in their houses so I could see the architecture and décor.

I pulled up on the street in front of the house, and was very confused. In front, a six-foot stone wall surrounded the property, about half an acre. A break in the front of it revealed a manicured stone semi-circle driveway, entering and exiting onto the street. It was gated, with an intercom.

A fountain nestled in the semi-circle inside the gate, and ivy and flowers that seemed to drip from it, trickling to the ground. Every blade of grass was the exact same height. I became nervous. Should I park in the driveway or on the street? He hadn't mentioned the gate or given me a code.

I was excited to see the house but now completely intimidated. What kind of person lived here? What did this person expect? Was I "the help"? Was I "an expert"? I was thinking too much. I did that a lot. I took a deep breath. *Be cool*, I thought. *He needs my help just like anyone else.* I relaxed into the fact that I had done this a thousand times before, and we all put our pants on one leg at a time.

I parked on the street. My nursing bag on my shoulder and

my cellphone and keys in my pocket, I headed for the electric gatekeeper. I pressed the intercom button.

"May I help you?" the voice asked.

"My name is Jessica. I'm the nurse here to see Mr. Ward," I said to it.

"Yes, come in. Mr. Ward is expecting you," it said.

The gate opened. There was no turning back. The front door was about twenty feet tall, or at least it seemed so to my five-foot-four-inch frame. Mr. Ward himself answered the door in his robe and motioned for me to come in, a cell phone clinging to his ear and mumbling some conversation.

It was cool inside. Outside the heat of the September day had just started to show. It had to be cool, I thought, because the foyer, which went on for days, was all solid marble. One step up was another central room with other halls and doors on their perimeters. Again, marble all through the floors met pillars at the four corners of the central room. It included the second level in its height, with a balcony surrounding the upper perimeter. Moldings were everywhere and somehow the neutral colors of the walls screamed extravagance because they were striped and swirled with navy and gold. A large plant or tree graced the center.

I had absorbed all of this in a few seconds while Mr. Ward, still embracing his cellphone, waved for me to follow him toward a room to the left. He was an average-looking man in his late fifties with a medium build, black hair and glasses. As I followed I glanced back, because I could, and out of the corner of my eye I saw an elevator. I guess we all had needs.

As he finished his call, he turned to me. "Hello. I'm sorry, I had to finish that call," he said. He was nervous and seemed distracted.

"That's okay," I responded. The room we entered seemed to be a den or study with deep red walls and stark white trim. I was unsure what he was doing until it became clear that this was where his supplies were. I was to change the dressing on his central IV line. But apparently there was a problem.

Mr. Ward explained, "I can't get this thing to work!" He stated nervously, "I have a meeting in an hour with my partners. They are coming here and I can't get this damn thing to work!" I knew his history and had my suspicions of what might be wrong.

Just then a woman appeared who shared his features. He introduced her as his sister.

"Would you like to do our visit here?" I asked, hoping there was a bathroom nearby to wash my hands. I then noticed there was a private bathroom door in the corner of the study. Silly me, to think this structure wouldn't be accommodating.

"No, we should probably go upstairs," he thought out loud. *Oh goody, the elevator!* I thought.

"Should we bring the supplies?" I suggested, and he agreed. His sister and another woman, a maid, helped to carry what I clearly could have lifted on my own.

The ride was fun, and I think he noticed my grin, although I tried to keep my poker-face on. It's the little things. I was concerned about his situation, though, and wished this moving of supplies had taken place prior to my coming, only for his lack of time, which seemed to be pressing, urgent even.

We entered a white room, the bedroom. The room was all white but for a stark teak wood four-poster California King bed and its brother-like highboy and sister bureau. Actually, I was discovering there were many different shades of white, and they were all adorably blended here, accented with incredible fresh floral arrangements on any surface that would hold them.

He lay himself back on a chaise, white fabric woven with gold, and opened his bathrobe. I now saw the problem. And I also saw my challenge in this lovely white room. Mr. Ward had what was called an ileostomy. He had his bowels resected and the small bowel diverted to exit through the abdominal wall. It is actually very common. The pouch containing the stool, which for people with ileostomies is very watery and acidic, kept coming loose. The acidity seeped under the adhesive wafer that kept the appliance stuck to the abdomen, causing it to loosen and leak. Well, leaking stool can be a concern.

At that moment I was grateful for my skills. It just so happened I was on the "Wound and Ostomy Team" and had specialized training in how to help this man, training that not all nurses had. I looked him in the eye and reassured him we could take care of this but would need someone to run to the medical supply store. "I can go!" his sister practically shouted. I gave her a shopping list: Eakin rings, ostomy cement, and a few more things. Off she went. The supply store was a convenient seven-minute drive from his house.

The maid went to get some towels and a washcloth and he relaxed some. And we began a conversation. "What line of work are you in?" I asked, trying to make him feel more normal. Okay, I also asked so I could find out what a person does for a living who lives like this.

"I'm in stocks, blah, blah, blah," he explained. It's not that I didn't listen; I honestly didn't understand a word he said. I smiled and he spoke a little more about his wife and their two children in New York and Phoenix. He asked what my husband did for a living, and I told him about the hardwood flooring business and that it was very small. "What is the name of his business?" he asked.

"Natural Hardwood Flooring," I replied. I loved the name. I told him how my sister and husband and I sat in a room, years before, and put ideas together for the name and how we came up with it. The name had changed, though, since the recession but at that time, it was the name. He was pleasant and it took his mind off the clock, I believe, to be distracted by the conversation.

I took his temperature, pulse and blood pressure and changed his central line IV dressing. I can't imagine how terrifying it would be for a non-medical layperson to have a leaking ileostomy, having asked for help before and found that help unsuccessful. I have had patients who had ceased going to church and the store and stop their lives because of this problem.

I loved that Mr. Ward was no longer a zip code to me. He was simply a man with a problem that I could do something about. So much of nursing is tasking, routine and simple. It's rarely like the drama of the television show *E.R.* Well, unless one works in the E.R., I guess! I would be lying, though, if I denied that a part of me loves being able to put on my hero's cape.

I know it sounds grotesque, but ileostomies never bothered me. Tracheostomy secretions and pus really bothered me. I know, how can anything bother a nurse?! Well, just ask one—we all have our Kryptonite! I almost vomited in front of a patient and surgeon one time when the surgeon did an incision and drainage at the patient's bedside and squeezed until most of the foul-smelling pus was out of the patient's leg wound. I felt my legs giving out under me and the room went dark and fuzzy. I held on to the patient's side-rail and handed the doctor 4X4 gauze as instructed until he was finished. Thank God for that side-rail! Anyway, poop doesn't bother me as much. And as a nurse I find it's very rewarding to have the skills to restore someone's dignity.

Mr. Ward's sister arrived in the nick of time with the supplies. I showed them how to warm and stretch the Eakin ring and wafer, to clean the stoma (the part of the intestine that comes through the skin), place the ring around it, then apply the appliance wafer and bag. He was to hold his hand against it for a while for warmth. He was to only use the cement under the ring if it was not lasting two days. The ring was resistant to the acidity of the stool. We got it all on and it looked as if it would work well. Time would tell, though, so I gave him some resources and more information should he continue to have problems.

Mr. Ward stood up. He straightened his back and the pouch stayed on. Peace came over his face. What a beautiful sight. He had five minutes. I packed my bags and followed him as he thanked me profusely. I accepted his thanks and told him I was glad he had a few minutes to spare to get dressed. He then began a line of questioning that confused me. "Do you like baseball?" he asked.

"It's okay," I said, not sure where this was going. He had things he needed to be doing.

"Do you like hockey?" he asked then, I began to get the idea.

"Well—" I started to reply.

"I know—football!" he said. I indicated a sort of yes, although I'm one of those rare St. Louisans who is not really into any sport. I did kind of like football, though. only because my grandfather used to take me to games and he explained everything, and it was a nice memory.

"Really, you don't need to," I said, realizing that he wanted to repay me somehow. There was also a rule, a BIG rule in the nursing profession, not to accept gifts, obviously, for ethical reasons. And they were not necessary anyway.

"I don't think you realize how grateful I am. They will be here any minute and it could have been a disaster," he persisted. I shook his hand.

"You're welcome, anytime," I said. It felt good to be appreciated.

"I have box seats for the Rams on October seventeenth. It's a Sunday," he continued.

"Really, Mr. Ward, we are not allowed to accept gifts," I uttered, sounding like a kid trying to follow the rules. "I'm sure your friends will be here soon." I began to make my way to the door.

I felt uncomfortable, I didn't want to be rude, but I did believe the wonderful gesture he was making was enough. I smiled and shook his hand, he returned the smile with a more relaxed smile as if he had just made a decision that pleased him. The maid met me and we descended via the elevator. I secretly said goodbye to the marble and pillars and stone and fountain, and went on with the day.

* * *

About two weeks later I was helping my husband by checking our business's P.O. box. I sometimes arrived home before him and those checks in the mail were always a good thing. I opened the box and found only a letter with no return address. I took it home and opened it.

It was two box-seat tickets to the Rams game on October seventeenth. That stinker! He had remembered the name of my husband's business, looked it up and mailed it to the address! How sweet was that!? We're not supposed to accept gifts. But who cares? We are rarely thanked for the work we do. Thanks are not necessary; it's our job. But it really does feel good! It feels good to be appreciated. Even seeing someone get better feels good. But this was a huge gesture.

As luck would have it, though, I was scheduled to work that day, which was okay with me. I ended up giving the tickets to my husband and his father, who enjoyed it immensely more than I would have. Accepting his sweet gift was somehow okay because I wouldn't use it. I could still enjoy the beautiful gesture through my husband and father-in-law. What lengths he had gone to! My job can be tedious, dirty, challenging, taxing, overwhelming and outright disgusting. Then every once in a while I realize that I can actually make a difference. What a powerful thing.

6

Michael

It was cold and overcast, about to rain or snow. It smelled fresh and wet at the same time, but with a stale under-wind. It matched my surroundings, I guess. I was in what some people in this city refer to as "the hood." When I pulled up to my patient's house, my tires crushed the Styrofoam cups and Snickers wrappers strewn about on the side of the dilapidated street.

I had to walk carefully up the four steps to the porch because a chunk of concrete had broken off and if left to habitual forward stair climbing, one could miss the faulty structure and take a nasty fall. The old red brick house had a tan/grey concrete porch. If one could look past the dirt and broken clay pots and cups and cigarette butts, one could barely see into the past.

When I tried, I saw a thriving, growing, proud area of North St. Louis, very much alive and hosting the 1904 World's Fair nearby, with guests from the far reaches of the earth. The address of the house in the film *Meet Me In St. Louis* was only blocks away. I envisioned a hot day with girls in corsets and big bonnets with bows being assisted by their gentlemen in tails and top hats out of horse-drawn carriages onto the concrete step, then the sidewalk. The concrete step was about ten inches high and a foot wide and three feet long. The steps were built at the curb, by the city, so the ladies wouldn't get their boots wet and would have an easy step down from their carriages. Many of those steps remain at the curb's edge today, in various spots in the city.

I saw hope. I saw the fruits of men's labors and dreams. I saw a hundred years of history of this mid-sized city as if it were all standing there at once. It now housed people who had given up, and a system that was broken. Those who still tried worked twice as hard as the ones who didn't, as if to scream that dignity and respect still lived there.

I rang the doorbell once. Twice. Then I knocked. Maybe the doorbell was broken. I couldn't remember. I had been there several times before; I had thought the doorbell worked, though. I had called him the night before, and he did answer and acknowledge the time for my visit. I knocked again. *Okay,* I thought. *Maybe I won't be doing the visit.*

I started to turn and the door opened. My patient, Michael, saw me and said nothing, opened the door wider and turned around yawning and sat down on his sagging couch. It was about 2:00 p.m. This day was unusual because he had guests, two female friends and one male. The ladies were dressed in brightly colored tank dresses that barely covered their nipples and buttocks. They walked to the front door and left. Still, no one had said a word.

"Hi, Michael," I said. He nodded and the other man went to the back room. "Can we get started?" Again, he nodded.

I smiled and set down my bag as a roach crawled out from under the couch. Michael had seen it and watched it crawl toward the kitchen. Up until now, it occurred to me that I had no fear. I had been doing nursing visits in some of the most crime-ridden areas of this city, which was one of the top five most dangerous cities in the country, for ten years. And I had no fear. I wondered why that was.

Are We Angels

A couch, a TV set on the floor, and a folding chair were the only pieces of furniture on the flat, dirty navy-blue rug. I picked up my bag and set it on the chair so the roach wouldn't get any ideas. I took Michael's temperature, blood pressure and pulse.

This visit was to be a courtesy visit for the doctor, who had requested we see this patient one more time to see what his excuse was for missing his third appointment with her. Michael had a serious foot wound from being diabetic. People with diabetes can lose feeling in their feet, and therefore can't always tell if something is lodged in one of them, or won't feel a painful wound.

He didn't take very good care of it. He also didn't manage his diabetes, despite all of the supplies and medicines being covered by Medicaid. Michael was basically what is termed a non-compliant patient. Medical professionals can only do so much in this situation. We can educate the patient and document the non-compliance. We had a saying: "You can't teach compliance." (The raw version was: "You can't fix stupid.")

So we were past the education stage and now at documentation. Michael wouldn't answer his phone for the doctor, so she wanted actual contact to give him the benefit of the doubt before she would refuse to continue his care because of non-compliance.

His foot dressing looked as if it hadn't been changed for days. "Michael, you need to be changing this dressing every day." My words fell on deaf ears. The nurse would assess the progress of the wound once a week. He was to do the dressing changes daily in between.

"Okay," he said to pacify me.

I put on my gloves. I unwrapped the dirty grey, dried-on green and yellow gauze that had once been white. It smelled. The wound was about two by five centimeters along the side of his foot, the size unchanged from last week. The bed of the wound was dark pink, with about thirty percent yellow slough and calloused edges. There was not much redness or swelling in the surrounding skin. I cleaned and redressed his foot. I always brought plastic grocery bags to pitch the dirty gauze because there were frequently no garbage liners in homes like these. I changed his PICC line dressing. As I worked, I began the line of questioning.

"Dr. Stone wants to know why you missed your last appointment with her this past Tuesday," I said, casually.

"I had an emergency."

Okay, I'll bite. "What was the emergency?"

"I had to help my roommate move," he said, with sincerity.

"Helping your roommate move is not an emergency," I said, but was about to be schooled.

"I had to help him move out because he shot someone, and the family of the guy he shot said they was gonna come here and get him and shoot up the place." *Oh my God.* I had a moment of denial at first, then a wave of panic swept over me like a surfer's tube. My heart pounded and everything got darker, or maybe it was the sun going behind a cloud. I became acutely aware of the noises outside and it became real to me that I was at that very moment in grave danger. I heard the man in the back room stir.

My limbs moved like lightning and my mind became laser clear, and as I threw my things back into my bag and slipped into my coat and dug for my keys, I rattled off to Michael the instructions. "Michael, we will no longer see you at this address. If you want we can see you at your sister's, but not again here."

He did not see the necessity of my actions, "No, it's okay. I put the word out in the 'hood that he moved out. No one's gonna come lookin' for him here."

"Michael," I said and turned and looked him in the eye,

putting my hand on his arm, "do you honestly think those guys are going to believe you? You need to leave. It's not safe for you here!" He just laughed and relaxed back into his cushions of denial. I, on the other hand, flew out the door and into my car, not feeling the steps and ground under my feet.

We got word about three days after my visit from one of our nurses who had taken a job in the E.R. at the main hospital. Michael had been stabbed seven times about the head and neck. He was dead on arrival. He was 37 years old.

7

Daisy

From my car I checked the front of the crumbled red brick house with the concrete porch, and around the sides of the house and street as far as I could see for any adult males who might be around, or any signs of danger. I was going to see another patient in my territory, in the city. I did a three-sixty looking all around. Nothing, again, only birds. The coast was clear. The hot sun glared relentlessly on my neck beneath my ponytail.

I exited the dark blue Jeep Cherokee that I loved. I felt safe in it, especially in the winter, with its four-wheel drive. From the trunk I grabbed the color-coded lab tubes, a lab requisition, lab bag, and some IV flushes. I knocked and Mrs. Price, the state-hired chore-worker, a dutiful, quiet woman in her mid-fifties, let me in.

"Hi, Mrs. Price." We exchanged smiles.

"Hello. Daisy is in the living room." It was her usual spot.

Daisy was a regular. I dreaded seeing her because she lacked manners. She was in her mid-seventies and had all the looks and all the charm of Jabba the Hutt. She had a mean streak. I had to be on guard with her while still fulfilling the role as the caring nurse. I was there to draw blood, change her central IV line dressing, and do wound care.

Are We Angels

Because we could wear street clothes in the field, I sometimes experimented. My outfit was not a good choice on that day, if I had wanted to avoid any commentary. I wore a thin cotton print peach top and khaki capri pants that kind of flared at the end and were not very flattering, but cooler in the stagnant, hot, humid St. Louis weather. Most of the homes I was to visit that day, including hers, had no air conditioning and I couldn't really wear shorts well. Sweat marks were already spreading under my arms.

Daisy's entire life was spent in that room. There was a hospital bed covered with dirty, stained sheets. The flat carpet was sticky. She walked only a few short steps each day to her throne, a bedside commode. She spent her whole day watching TV and napping. The house smelled of stool, bacon and Lysol, Mrs. Price's attempt at providing some sense of order in the house.

"You're kinda heavy, aren't you?" Daisy said, her four-hundred-plus-pound body leaning over slightly, eyes riveting into mine, as if sharing a secret with me. I tried not to show the utter shock, disappointment, and embarrassment I'd just experienced. After all, she's merely making conversation. *I under-weigh her by more than half!* I thought, completely self-consciously. Moments like these allowed me to refine my poker face. I've mastered it over the years.

"Daisy, that's not very nice to say," I said aloud. Correcting a seventy-five-year-old woman on her manners was apparently also part of my job. Her job was to get a rise out of me. What else was there for her to do? This home-nurse thing was marvelous entertainment. I helped her. She shocked me. It was a win-win situation.

Dogs barking in the background alerted my peripheral senses and I paid attention as I continued my work. Mrs. Price was cleaning in the kitchen and it felt good to have her present, in case things got out of hand. "How are you feeling today?" I began again with Daisy, swatting a fly away and trying to make light.

"I ache all over in my back and I didn't move my bowels for three days but now they're going good," she said releasing a large flatulence from under her on her throne.

"Good," I said, knowing how she loved to discuss her bowels. "Is your pain medicine working?"

Rawf, Rawf! We heard deep loud barking outside of the opaque window.

She nodded. "Those damn dogs, always barking! I got to turn the TV up to drown them out every damn day." She leaned in again, and shared another secret. "I asked that woman the other day why she got those damn dogs and she said so they can lick her," she confided. Again, making conversation. My shock-o-meter was a little overwhelmed this time. *Was this really true?* I thought. Damn; she was in my head again.

"Daisy, really!" I said, acknowledging this time that she had crossed the line. It made me wonder, though, if all nightmares really do come true, somewhere. *As The World Turns* was on the TV and provided a good distraction for us, as it usually did, a peaceful relief from those awkward conversations. This was even one of her lighter conversation days.

I finished drawing labs and doing IV line care. A peek out the window reassured me that my beloved Jeep was untouched. I reached into the paper bag containing the wound supplies.

Hers were not actually wounds. Daisy had elephantiasis of the legs. This swelling condition left her legs and feet huge and swollen like an elephant's, with thick, ruddy, grey, scaly skin. There were deep valleys between the toes and where the skin swelled and folded over the ankles. It can be caused by worms that infest the lymph system in the body, or untreated lymphedema, or swelling from problems with the lymphatic system, usually from certain cancer treatments. She had survived cancer but had not complied with the lymphedema treatment. The care included washing her legs, then applying a special four-layer wrap that went from foot to knee, three times a week.

It was Monday, and the wraps had been on since Friday. Daisy said that they itched. I got a pan of warm water, soap, a washcloth and towel from Mrs. Price. The outer layer was Coban, which is like ace wrap except it is sticky, and I cut it off easily. The next layer was off-white, ace-like compression wrap. Next was a cream-colored tight wrap. The last was a layer of cotton wrap. As I unwrapped the last layers, I noticed the white cotton layer down by her toes was brown. This was unusual. I unwrapped from the knee down. I was, at this point, covered in sweat.

"Did you spill some coffee on your feet?" I asked, unwrapping the cotton.

"No," she replied, the inflection going up at the end of her syllable.

"Did someone spray something around the floor?" I prodded, wondering where this brown color came from.

"No," she again replied. Mrs. Price peeked around from inside of the kitchen. I unwrapped the ankle and the foot, around and around, then the toes.

"There's brown stuff down by your toes on the cotton layer of your wraps."

The windows were covered with blankets to keep the heat out. The darkness of the room forced me to lean in to see. I unraveled the cotton down to her feet. When I removed the cotton completely it became clear. I jumped back, letting out an audible gasp. They were white against her dark and grey skin, some of them stuck in the folds. Dozens of them, with their squiggling little bodies. I dropped the cotton wrap and began to breathe heavily. I froze and stared. I could not move.

"What is it?" Daisy asked, a tremble in her voice. I could not speak. I tried to, I had to. How would I tell her? How could I say these words? But I was a professional! A professional what? Oh, yeah, a nurse.

It must have been a loud shriek because Mrs. Price walked

in, "Damn, Daisy! You got maggots on your foot!" She had such a way with words. *Thank you, Mrs. Price!* I thought. Her words helped kick me out of a frozen state. Now it was out there. I was able to assume the role of the caregiver again.

"It's going to be okay," I told her. Her head hung even lower than it usually did and to the side, as if to hide. The skin on her face had fallen. How embarrassed she was! She knew she was a mess, but this was too much, even for her.

I couldn't stand how this was making her feel. Instantly I knew what to do and who I was in all this. I had to get the maggots off. I got the pan of water and put on two sets of gloves. I put her first foot in the water. They didn't come off willingly. I had to push their little squiggling bodies out from between her toes, and from under the skin folds. (If you aren't puking by now, you might consider a career in the medical profession.)

My shoulder was cradling my cellphone as I pried away the last of them. I saved a few and put them in a sterile specimen container. Daisy's face was that of a scared child now. Embarrassment overwhelmed her. Thank God for Mrs. Price. "All it takes is one fly. Just one. Mmmm, mmm." She shook her head. She looked at me with a mixture of thankfulness and I'm-glad-I-don't-have-your-job on her face. "We're gonna have to clean some more around the room here."

I spoke with the doctor who said she should be fine but for her to go to the E.R. just in case. I stayed with her until the ambulance came. I sent the specimen cup as well, and Mrs. Price and I reassured her as the responders heaved her onto a stretcher and took her away. I told my supervisor. Apparently, maggots were used years ago for wound debridement, or removal of dead tissue. I thanked Mrs. Price and went on to my next patient. And on my way home, I stopped by Walgreens and bought a fly swatter.

8

The Bell

A gold-plated eight-inch bell on a walnut plaque had a large paper clip attached to the clapper to extend it and allow the clapper to hit the inside for a clear *DING*! It hung like a sconce on the wall of the cancer center, near the check-in desk. A gold plate below it read, "Donated by Mr. and Mrs. Steinhurst. He who rings this bell rings it in celebration, for his chemo is done and his cancer is gone." It was a beautiful bell. It was a celebration bell. This is a story of one of the rings of the bell.

* * *

Let me begin by describing the cancer center and a notoriously memorable day. The pressure was on. I was working at the cancer center for home infusion. I worked with Kim along-side the cancer-center nurses. Patients receive two to four hours of chemotherapy at the cancer center. Our job was to hook patients to a chemotherapy pump that they would go home with for two days. A home infusion nurse would then be sent to the patient's house to disconnect the pump.

It was an impossibly busy day. Twenty patients were scheduled for hook-up that day and Kim and I were scrambling. A normal day was five to six patients each.

"It looks like there were some schedule changes as well as some new patients. I guess nobody informed us. We are going to need some help," I said, when I phoned our office. Somehow I knew my request would be rejected.

"We had a call-in and everyone's full," Renee explained. Renee, another nurse, did staffing at the home infusion office a few miles away. I didn't believe what she said was true. I had worked in the field. I could have easily run by the cancer center to help after seeing four to five patients in their homes, and I had on several occasions. That's probably how I ended up working there three days a week. Kim was there full time. She was my mentor. She was the swan and I was like a big clumsy dog, but I was learning.

"There will probably be some cancellations, won't there?" Renee said.

When a patient is scheduled for treatment but the lab-test results from a blood draw beforehand indicates that treatment isn't safe yet, the treatment would have to wait a week, or until another intervention is done so they can tolerate their chemotherapy. On that day, though, everyone was ready. Renee also knew that we wouldn't find out whether there were any cancellations until it was too late. It was pointless. We stopped trying to ask after a few months there. It was what it was.

"Let us know if anyone can help later," I stated, and hung up. I began to prepare myself mentally for the monster day.

"I can do this," I said to myself aloud, and breathed in, then out. "Kim, let's split these patients up. We can do this!"

Kim looked at me blankly. She had been at this for years, longer than I. I was her only real help and there only three days a week. She took a long breath and said something that changed forever the way I viewed my career. "Yeah, we can do this. But why would anyone *want* to?" Her words hit me like a burst of wind, nearly knocking me off of my feet. Why is it that we nurses pride ourselves on our ability to tolerate impractical, unattainable challenges?

I paused. Why, indeed? Why would anyone want to be heroes, be fast, be tough, be strong, be short-handed, be needlessly rushed, neglected, used, told over and over that there's no help. Why be told "no," when the respectful, honest thing would be to say to the nurse, "Hey, we're short-handed today. Can we ask that you go that extra mile?" In this case they wouldn't ask. Because a question like that implies a problem. And a problem requires a solution. And why have a solution when nurses are there and would do twice the work for the same amount of pay? For months, years? We hadn't agreed to this.

Kim rolled her eyes. Our hearts pumped with anxiety and I rolled my eyes, too. We put on our 'show smiles' and dug in. We had no choice.

"You know how we talked about opening that little dress shop?"

"Come on!" I said, and pulled her arm, dragging her into the chemo pods.

We were employees of the hospital, not the university/cancer center. Only the cancer center nurses were employees, so there was no sharing of computer systems. Even the FBI and CIA can share information these days, but unfortunately one of the best cancer centers in the Midwest cannot. It even seemed silly for our jobs to exist. The cancer center nurses could easily hook up the patient to the home chemo pump, but a crisscross in billing somewhere and legalities made it so we, the home infusion nurses, had to do it. And I was glad. On normal days I loved it. What I wanted was to learn and practice the skills needed for this job, and be there for the patients, if they wanted to talk.

Kim and I took patients by turn as each came in. They were first taken to an elongated white room with chairs and counters covered with test tubes, port access kits, saline syringes, alcohol wipes and a window through a wall into a room that was the lab. Most of the patients had ports, miniature hockey puck-like devices with rubber tops. A port's tail goes into a major vein. It is surgically implanted under the skin and accessed with a needle that can remain in use for up to a week. Half of the patients would see the doctor. All would have their ports accessed and get their blood drawn from their port by either the cancer center nurses or by us. The blood was given to the lab which delivered results in minutes.

Chemo can make white and red blood cells and platelet levels go down. The cells are expected to go down, then come back up a few weeks after a chemo dose. If the levels did not come back up enough, the patient might not be able to get their next cycle of chemo. This is bad. People want their chemo. It kills their cancer.

Kim and I waited for lab results and if it was a "go", meaning the levels were acceptable, began our scramble. Because of the system, and the lab's employees belonged to a different system than ours, we had to wait for the doctors' handwritten orders. Simply making a copy was not an option, I guess. Not every patient of the cancer center would get home chemo, so their nurses didn't always look out for which patient was which. They just needed to get their portion started. So we would chase the cancer center nurses around for the paper orders and try to catch them before they'd give them to their pharmacy down the hall where the paper orders would be stuck for a crucial twenty to forty minutes until the pharmacy was done mixing the chemo.

If we didn't catch the orders from their nurses (occasionally they faxed the orders to our home care pharmacy for us) our patients would be stuck there, waiting. Our homecare pharmacists, several miles away, needed a two-hour turnaround between a faxed paper order and delivery of the chemo and pump at any one of four random drop-off places in the building. Which one depended on the courier/driver that day.

Are We Angels

The cancer center nurses were busy too, trying to get everyone started with their pre-medications, drugs given before chemo to prevent side effects, and checking everything. Good nurses check formulas and mathematical calculations for chemo drugs before giving them. Yes, doctors make mistakes, rarely. Nurses are the last to check medications and are responsible for giving the patients the right drugs and doses at correct times and rates.

Kim and I swarmed around the cancer center nurses, trying to stay out of their way. Our biggest challenge was to look completely cool and stress-free. Cancer patients don't need more stress. They don't want to be there. They went because they had to; it was their job. Well, it was more like community service: a few torturous hours every couple of weeks. They didn't need more stress and they didn't like to wait.

This cancer center was beautiful, though, with four large rooms called pods and six chairs, and a private enclosed room in each pod. Between each pod was a sitting area with restrooms and a kitchen usually adorned with fresh homemade goodies that patients' families brought in for each other and the staff. Comfort foods were big there.

All the way around the exterior walls of the pods and kitchens were continuous large windows revealing the park behind the building: A vibrant garden, with winding sidewalks and arbors dripping with greenery and flowers. Patients were in leather recliner chairs about six feet apart, exposed to each other, yet with an invisible cushion of air space. Some talked and shared and laughed and cried with each other. Others withdrew into their own little worlds of novels and earbuds.

The cancer center nurses were mostly young, bubbly and oozing with stories of boyfriends, diets, iPhones, and family members with cancer. I think they gave the patients hope. I think they were selected for their youth, their freshness and sweetness.

There were many faces. The cancer center's business grew by logarithms. When I started there, they didn't fill two pods on any given day. Two years later they could barely contain them in four. Business, unfortunately, was that good. Our home infusion staff had never increased, though, despite the growth.

I was working, personally, on my own stress level, feeling frequently overwhelmed by my job. I loved working with these special patients, but I hated the lack of help and resources. I was married with three boys under age eight. Although I loved my work, I frequently worked fifty, sixty, seventy hours a week. I worked at the cancer centers three days a week, then in the field two days, including weekends and evening/night on-call. The computer work was an infinite spiral of never-ending drag: Thirty to forty pages or so for a new admission (the number of pages had actually been reduced), to ten to fifteen for each patient seen that day, to recertification computer work, every two months, and ongoing on each of the fifty or so patients we each managed. I had not signed up for that lifestyle. It crept up on me, like my twenty-pound weight gain. I felt like a perpetually unavailable mom.

Our office was several miles away, and the boss never came to check on us or see what needed tending from a supervisor's perspective. I'm not sure what was really going on, but she entered her office in the morning and left at the end of the day. Nothing was managed. I don't know whether her hands were tied, or if she had major depression, or what was going on. We couldn't keep new nurses. We lost about five that year. They quit after a few weeks, citing a "toxic environment." We felt neglected, and while we managed ourselves, whenever we asked for help or other solutions to situations, we were told no. Procedural problems were neglected. Staffing was neglected. The system was poorly managed. It was a sinking ship.

It had gotten so bad at one point that despite our scrambling and doing everything correctly a patient once cursed me and the place I worked for. He walked out back to the garden and cried because his home chemo still hadn't arrived from our home care pharmacy two hours after the cancer-center chemo was done.

"You mean to tell me you've had two and a half hours and your office still can't get my chemo here for another hour? What the hell is the hold-up? I need to get home; my wife has to get back to work!"

"I'm so sorry, sir. I really apologize. I wish there was something that I could do. I know you have other things to do. I will keep checking on it for you and let you know as soon as it gets here." I could only eat crow, take one for the team that is so faithful to Kim and me. Overcome with medication induced moodiness, stress, and a legitimate complaint, he walked to the back of the garden and cried. I wanted to go back there and cry with him.

Instead, I did my own commiserating with God. He and I grew close during this time. I needed this job. I would keep trying to manage better. I kept looking for ways I could work better or more efficiently. I was chronically stressed. But I loved working there. I saw love and hope in places I never knew existed, and saw very sick, desperate patients that seemed to have already allowed the cancer to eat their souls. Only the body's shell remained. I cared about these people. I wanted to do right by them. They deserved the best we could give.

I knew this wouldn't last forever. I was not cut out for a continuously high-stress job. But I wasn't ready to let it go. In the future, I wrote the name of this job on a piece of paper and buried it during a letting-go-of-things-that-are-killing-you ceremony, with my husband's nudging. God would quickly respond with the next phase of my work. But until then—

On this day it was my turn to stay late. Kim and I always worked out which of us came early and which one stayed late. All we had was each other. She had become a trusted friend and mentor. She had a way of seeing through the mess to what was important. We worked well together. Five to six hookups to home chemo was normal; we each had about ten. But we made it through. It was a miracle no hook-ups were late. And then *she* came: Sandy, the 4:00 appointment that finished by 6:00. Like clockwork, she was always on time.

Sandy didn't look like a patient. She came after work. She ran a hotel. Very tall and thin, she had golden-brown straight hair that lay elegantly to just below her jaw and flipped outward ever so slightly. She had a long rectangular face and wore long straight skirts, and scarves, and bangles, and always a smile. It was all business to her and she was here to get her job done.

She was a regular, a lifer. Her cancer was such that she needed chemo for the rest of her life, a requirement she accepted gracefully, dutifully, despite rocking a seventy-hour work week, every week. What a woman!

A few months before, I had disconnected her chemo and had to visit her, of course, at her workplace. In the hotel lobby, about ten guests were in line and waiting around. I felt as if I drew far too much attention with my stethoscope around my neck, my name badge, and toting my huge blue nursing bag which could not be mistaken for luggage. All eyes were on me. I detested that with a vengeance. I asked at the front desk for Sandy.

"Who shall I say is here for her?" asked a man with an upturned nose, stiff posture, perfectly cut light hair and a suit and tie.

"Jessica. Sandy's expecting me." Sandy knew who I was. If he needed to know more he could look at my name badge.

"I'll let her know you're here." He picked up the phone. After a brief exchange he said, "Sandy will be a few minutes. You can wait here or by her office."

"Where is her office?" I wanted to be anywhere but in front of those gawking eyes. *I'm a professional, stop being so proud,* I thought. Grudgingly I gave the man a fake smile while he gave me a series of unclear directions and I went on to figure out the maze. At least there weren't any more onlookers.

A stealthy map-reader, I have a knack for finding things and was relieved to find her office quickly. There was a waiting area and gratefully I sat down. I could hear her talking on the phone to someone in her office at the same time. Proactively she trouble-shot, streamlined, problem-solved, and delegated her way to the next task, which was her chemo. I felt dizzy watching her.

As gracefully as a ballerina she gestured for me to come in.

"Hi. You look busy!" I said, wrapping the blood pressure cuff around her outstretched arm. She knew the routine. Thermometer in her mouth, 98.2 F, and pulse taken.

"Is it finished?" I asked.

"Yes, the pump beeped a few minutes ago and I turned it off. We are so short-handed. One of my best managers moved to another state and we've all been filling in." She let her guard down a little. "It's been crazy! And it's been four months now. Corporate is supposed to be filling this position but it seems to be taking forever. So, it's been seventy-hour work weeks for me." She smiled a fake smile. I know those well.

I removed the chemo tubing from the pump and disconnected it from her port tube, stuffing it into a special chemo disposal bag. "That's an awful lot for you, Sandy," I said. "Are you feeling okay? Any nausea? Diarrhea?" I rubbed her port tip with alcohol and flushed it with saline, pulling back halfway for only a second to make sure there was a blood return, then flushed the rest in.

"No, I actually feel fine. I know it's strange," she laughed at my perplexed expression. "I drink about two liters of water a day and I'm always moving. That's probably got a lot to do with it." I shook my head. I then flushed the port with heparin, pulled all of the clear tape-like dressing up around the special needle. She stiffened her back and turned her head and I held the skin beneath her port tightly against her chest and with the other hand pulled the needle out. We finished with a two by two inch gauze and tape.

"I'm sure that has a lot to do with it," I said. "But you're still amazing! I barely handle my fifty- or sixty-hour weeks and I'm not going through chemo!" Quickly I packed my bag and she stood up with me to say goodbye.

"I sure hope they find someone soon, Sandy," I said. She smiled a smile that looked like a wish.

"Me, too," she said. "See you next time." She rolled her eyes.

"Yes, see you then."

That had been months before. Back at the cancer center, Sandy set her bags down, brushed her hair out of her eyes and smoothed her grey skirt. Her port accessed, blood work done, she was a "go."

She smiled. "Hi! How are you?" She did it like clockwork. Get lab work: check. Get pre-medications: check. Get chemo: check. I wondered how she remained calm and beautiful during her treatments. I felt like a slug by comparison. Why couldn't I be so calm despite my non-cancer life stressors? *Oh, yeah, that's what the poker face is for.*

"I'm fine. How's the hotel?" I said as I eyeballed Jen, a cancer-center nurse, who almost ran the orders to their pharmacy in haste, but raised her finger as she caught my eye, indicating she would fax them to home care's pharmacy first. *"Thanks, Jen,"* I mouthed from across the room.

"Still looking for that manager," Sandy said. I gave her an empathetic look. "It wouldn't be so bad, but my husband and I were planning on a trip to Las Vegas in two weeks." She slowed down and let out a sigh. "We have to cancel."

"No!" I was truly saddened for her. Then, while she was venting, something in my gut said *Pray for her.* Well, that was unexpected! I hadn't even been thinking anything remotely like that. My thoughts had been on salvaging her Vegas trip. She was still talking so my sudden thought didn't register on my face. And I had a great poker face.

Strange as the feeling was, I went with it. I nodded, still listening externally, but switched on my mental tape recorder so I could rewind it and replay it at any time if quizzed. And in the foreground of my mind I thought, *Sandy is whole and healed, no more cancer.* Great, these secret little prayers. No one has to know. I told her how sad I was for her that she had to cancel her trip. She vented but then said they held out hope for another trip, and so on and so on. She was delightful.

A few weeks later I was the "late" nurse again. I let Kim go early and took advantage of the time spent waiting for Sandy's arrival by trying to catch up on computer work that was about two weeks behind. Ugh! A little more than half of the employees had left for the day. Most of the patients were gone except for one or two. I set up my laptop and papers in a cubby-like area in the hall, with a clear view of the front doors in case a lost-looking courier came in with a box of chemo and its pump.

While chipping away at the glacier of work in front of me, deep in thought, with nothing but peace in the hallway, I heard a *DING*!!! One clear, loud *ding* from the bell. I nearly jumped out of my skin! My fingers and toes felt aftershocks. *Who could that be?* I wondered. *And why didn't anyone come get me to celebrate with them?* They actually did that. They would gather as many people as possible to celebrate with the patient about to ring the bell. Only Mr. Meyer and that other lady were back in the pods. *Who could that be?*

Then I heard a woman's sobs. They got louder and I heard two sets of footsteps. Then I saw Sandy and her husband walking up the hall. He was tall as well, built like a big bear with kind brown eyes. Sandy was sobbing uncontrollably, his arm tight around her thin shoulders. I came out from inside the cubby into the hall.

"Sandy, did you ring the bell?" I asked, puzzled. This made no sense.

"Yes," she sobbed. She must have just seen her oncologist. "The doctor said no more chemo. I am cancer-free!" She grabbed me and hugged me, and I hugged her back, trying to wrap my brain around this miracle. She was a lifer. She had to have chemo for life. All of the craziness of my life and that job stopped and stood still. She was cancer free? I didn't know how this was possible, and HIPAA wouldn't allow me to find out. What I was witnessing there was a miracle. Like, a miracle, for real.

Then it hit me: the prayer! *Did my prayer have something to do with this? Nah. Maybe. Wow!! No way. Ok, whatever. No. Maybe?!* I was shocked. I don't claim to have any "gifts" or "powers" at all. I don't really believe in "faith healings" and I'm not particularly religious. I know it wasn't me. But I felt completely humbled. Like, stupid-happy. I felt like one of those toy circus monkeys clapping his cymbals together with a stupid grin on his face, saying, *Wow, God, that was amazing, again! Again! Do it again!"* I didn't really care how it happened. It just happened.

I watched in awe. Frozen. Given over to whatever this was. I couldn't move a muscle. I simply enjoyed it. I was filled with happiness for her. Then just as suddenly as she had appeared, she and her husband walked away through the glass doors, out into the sunset, into their happily-ever-after. I guess stories like these were the reason I stayed so long at that job.

9

Quitting

I feel as if I go to a dark place when I complain in stories like these. I hear a voice from my childhood saying, "you can do it," and "never complain about too much work," and "nurses are tough, they can take it." I wondered why I couldn't take it anymore. I didn't have a black foot! I didn't have cancer! Who the hell was I to complain? I felt I had no right. I shut myself up before I even started, and would stew because I was still so unhappy.

Why not just get another job? There were many reasons. For starters, I'm a slow learner. I tend to learn things slowly and completely, and to be an absent-minded perfectionist. I couldn't stand the thought of learning a whole new job at that point. I didn't have it in me. I had a lot of personal stress. We lost our house in the recession. My husband's flooring business had tanked. I used to run the business and also worked several days a month for home infusion. I had gone back to nursing full time. We needed health insurance. We needed money. My husband scrambled every day trying to restart another business without any help. We had three boys, ages eight, five and three years old.

For years I went into neighborhoods in St. Louis wracked

with crime and poverty. I was a tough girl. I had nursed my boys as babies, pulled into the parking lots of churches between seeing patients in these areas, locked the car doors, covered the windows with towels and pumped my milk for them. I was fearless, brave. But something happened during this time, after my third son came along.

A picture was forming in my mind like that of a subtle dark mystery or horror film. I was no longer brave. I found myself in the middle of this life, and slowly over time, as the workload increased, I became tired. I wanted to be a good mom. This was my top priority. Yet my life did not reflect this.

All of my complaints might have sounded as if I was selfish. Self-care seemed so foreign to me, like a dirty word. I had no boundaries. I felt a deep painful guilt that sat like a heavy meal in my stomach with palpable nausea from the thought that being a nurse was killing me. I had grown to hate my job, yet was completely dependent on it. The guilt swelled in my gut. I was never home and if I was, it would be, "No, baby, not now. Ask Daddy," or "I can't! I have three hours of computer work to do!" And full of annoyance, mainly because I couldn't be the mom I wanted to be, I sat on the couch, unapproachable, and worked. I was no longer tough. I was tired, exhausted. I felt as if everyone wanted a piece of me. I was falling through a tunnel of my own hell, because although I had a wonderful family I could not be there for them and enjoy them.

I could not live up to the image of the all-angelic, sweet, receptive nurse anymore. I didn't have time. I wanted to help people, to be kind, but the overwhelming work consumed me. My job always seemed to want more from me. More, more, more. I couldn't have a decent conversation with a patient because of time. Then at home I tried to be the best mom I could be. But I had no time. Sometimes I shut the computer off and spent time with my family. Then Monday, I received emails asking where my work was at. *Screw them and their f***ing* *computer work!* I thought. *I'm spending time with my kids!* I stole time. I became a thief of time. And because I knew it was wrong no matter what I did—neglect my kids or neglect my computer work—I lived in a constant state of guilt.

I tried to focus on what I had. I consciously made myself feel grateful. I did have a job. Many people didn't. I had a supportive, hard-working husband. Many women didn't. We had children; many people could not have them. It was a constant battle to talk myself out of a severe depression. I could not afford depression. We had people depending on us. *I am grateful, I am grateful.*

Eventually, that job worsened. I can't really describe it here, but let's just say certain people skirted the rules and I was backed into a corner, forced to "take out insurance" to protect myself. I am no longer naïve. The last year there I was the only nurse there able to "fill in" on every job: visits in the field, the infusion suites in the office, and all four of the cancer centers we served. I was on the committee and re-wrote the patients' infusion teaching sheets with the help of some co-workers. I was on the wound-ostomy team. I could do it all, and did it well. And I never lost sight of the main reason we were there: the patients. I was proud of that. They were, after all, what it was all about.

Whether it was administration, management, a broken internal system or our broken national system of healthcare, I don't know, but the issue reached a boiling point. That last year they changed the pay from hourly to salary. Seven nurses and three supervisors quit or were fired. After fifteen years there, and I would have stayed there indefinitely, I found another job and finally quit.

10

Sleepover

I love working the holidays! Just kidding. I would be lying if I said it was a life goal of mine to have a job requiring me to work a varied selection of 24/7 hours, 365 days a year. Who works when the weather turns dangerous? While schools, churches, airlines, businesses, and retail stores may close, gas station employees, grocery store workers, police and fire people, restaurant workers, and health care facilities are always open. (I'm sure I've missed some professions, apologies to you!) Since the beginning of my career I have worked nights, evenings, weekends, birthdays, president's days, mother's days, father's days, summers, and holidays. I have worked them all.

Nurses know this when they sign up for this life. It's a sacrifice we make. Many a Christmas or Thanksgiving I've awoken at 5:00 a.m., a bit resentful about the peaceful, snow-covered streets not lined with drivers because they are in their safe, cozy houses, at rest. Some brilliant hospitals in the 1970s came up with the idea of twelve-hour shifts to attract and retain nurses during the nursing shortage. Twelve hours of constant running to ease pain and suffering, and interruptions during tedious tasks can be life-draining, but I admit I loved the hours. If full-time is what you need, it's the best deal around. Usually shifts are not worked in a row, although some nurses prefer this. The dangling, effective carrot is that the nurse is off for four days every week.

The other carrot is the numerous roles nurses can fulfill. Nurses can work in hospitals, outpatient facilities, home care, schools, clinics, prisons, military bases, camps, parishes, industrial facilities, insurance companies, cruise ships, and triage or help phone lines such as crisis or poison-control centers. There's also legal nursing, quality-control nursing, nursing educators, research nursing, pharmaceutical and equipment sales nursing, nurse/midwifery, forensic nursing, nurse anesthetist, wound ostomy nursing, nursing IT professionals, nurse managers, FEMA, Salvation Army, Peace Corps and Red Cross nursing, and the newer exciting field of nursing informatics, to name a few. So many carrots, and so many ways to be of service. Also you are allowed to work in your pajamas (scrubs).

It was New Year's Day. My mood was sour, with a Barbie Doll smile plastered on my face to hide my true angst. I was new to the hospital. I had been there for about a month, fresh out of orientation. I was a bit backward in how I sequenced my career. I worked at Children's Hospital first, then pediatric home care and private duty, then adult private duty, adult home care, home infusion, and then the adult hospital.

My organization and computer documentation skills were raw and slow. I needed to learn. I swallowed my insecurity and put one foot in front of the other through the parking lot toward the automatic double doors that led past the E.R. to the elevators. A heavy snowstorm was predicted. I was scheduled to work the next two days. The snow would start midday and continue all night, heavy and with accumulation to six inches expected by nightfall, with two to six more inches to fall that night. For Minnesotans or Canadians, that is merely a dusting. But in St. Louis everything closes; the city shuts down.

My shoulder ached as the heavy overnight bag's strap pulled downward. I had a hard time packing light. My husband and I had discussed it. I planned on staying overnight at the hospital. He felt better knowing I was safe. I didn't like risking the drive in the snow. My minivan once got stuck in snow, when I had done home care, and the resultant cold, waiting, and concern for my husband who braved to snow to come dig me out, was not good. I had kissed my boys goodnight the night before and encouraged them to have fun raiding the kitchen and playing video games while being snowed in.

We nurses needed to be there. My boss had called everyone scheduled to work during the snowstorm. "You know, it is expected that you work your shift," Peggy said, as tactfully as she could.

"Yes, I know. I plan on sleeping over," I said.

"Oh boy, that sounds fun," she said sarcastically. "Christy will help you tonight with the sleeping arrangements once the house supervisors figure out how many are staying. You can check with her, okay?"

"What happens if someone gets stuck in the snow?"

"They have a couple of people ready with four-wheel-drive vehicles who can go out and help people if they need it."

"That's good. Thanks." I said. I wondered what people had done before cellphones. I thought back to my early home care days. We simply knocked on strangers' doors and waited longer.

The elevator ascended to the fifth floor. I left my overnight bag in the locked conference room and went to my locker. I started my day.

Some nurses opted to stay at a nearby hotel. Some nurses lived nearby. Some had trucks. I lived about twelve minutes from work, two towns over, but didn't want to take any chances on the hilly highway in my minivan. So I went to work, a freshman embarking on two twelve-hour shifts as a blizzard approached.

Are We Angels

We worked through the first shift. It was the weekend. We watched from our fifth-floor tower as the dark clouds came in and littered cotton balls as far as the eye could see, leaving a piled-up thick white blanket of snow over the hills and stick-figured trees, a view that was silent and breathtaking. I was still new and trying to find my organization and pace, and didn't finish until late. I didn't yet know anyone really well, and everyone from our floor had gone, risking it on the roads.

Our supervisor counted who was staying and who wasn't, and left earlier in the afternoon. The next floor over, our sister floor's supervisor Christy stayed, according to their plan for extended working during the storm. It was about 8:20 p.m., 20:20 hours. I was exhausted and a little uncomfortable about sleeping over.

I wanted to be one of those office workers allowed to stay home, to hang out with my husband and kids and play games and bake cookies and warm myself by the fire. But I was there. My husband and kids were fine. I called them and gave them my love. I hid the longing I felt to be with them, and again used my brave voice.

Another nurse, a dark-haired woman named Rose from our sister floor, was in the break room when I walked in. "Are you staying, too?" I asked.

"Yes," she said. "Do you know where we are supposed to go?" I hadn't even thought of that yet. I was late finishing and so was she.

"No," I replied. No one else was around. They must all have been given their places to sleep. "I guess we should check with Christy?"

We walked across the hall to her office. "I was told you should talk to the house supervisor," Christy said with a smile. She looked tired, too.

We phoned the "House Sup," as she was called, and were instructed to go to conference room C. Loading up our bags and pillows we dragged them onto the elevator down to the ground floor. The exterior walls of our hospital were all glass, and the snow was then about calf-height with more falling each hour.

Curious family members passed us in the hall and chuckled at how we looked in our scrubs, dragging all of our stuff. We arrived at conference room C: a bunch of cots in a big conference room. Rose and I dropped our stuff by the door. We looked all around for open cots, but all were taken! There was either a woman sleeping already or a name on a piece of paper on each cot. *Surely this couldn't be true*, I thought. Our supervisors would have planned for us; after all, earlier that day we had given them our names. Surely this was a mistake.

Discouraged, tired, hungry and loaded with stuff, we left. "What should we do?" I asked Rose, rhetorically.

"I don't know." She was equally exhausted. "I guess we could call the house supervisor. But I'm worried. What if there's not enough room for us?"

"I would hope not!"

We stood outside for a minute discussing what to do, enthusiastic as weak kittens. It was dark. The cotton balls continued to fall. Rose then glanced over and her body followed her eyes to the next conference room with a whole bunch of empty cots!! We dragged our stuff over and plopped our bundles onto two empty cots, and grabbed our purses.

Now that we had found our haven, we were off to find a quick bite to eat. We headed upstairs to the wonderful little coffee shop that also served soup and pizza and sandwiches. We grabbed some sandwiches and salads and juice and found a quiet spot.

Rose told me she was from China.

"How long have you been in the U.S.?"

"About six years. Things are so different here. I'm still getting used to it," she said. She used no dressing on her salad. I drowned mine in Ranch. One of the differences was food, it seems.

"We abuse our vegetables. I can see that difference," I joked.

"Yes, it's just a cultural thing, I think."

"Do you have family here?"

"Yes, a husband and five-year-old boy."

"I have a husband and three boys. It's hard to leave them like this, isn't it?"

"But they're fine."

"I think it's harder on us than it is them!" It always was, I thought. I was only trying to make light of the mood I was in.

When we finished, we went back to our cots. We were the only people there. While I was pulling leggings and a T-shirt and a toothbrush out of my bag, Rose waved her hand and said in a worried voice, "Did you see those papers?"

I had not. On each of the other cots was a quarter-sheet of paper with writing on it. As we looked closer, we read: "Michael", "Tyrone", "Chris", "Joe."

I was so tired my contact lenses felt like sandpaper. My legs and feet ached, and for a split second I actually thought, how bad could it be, sleeping in a room with a bunch of strange men? Then a voice inside said *Hell no!* I was sure they were nice men and all, but, no thanks. Rose felt the same. We were back to square one. We called Christy. She was no longer in her office. Then we called the House Sup.

"I thought you went to conference room C," she said.

"Conference room C was full," I said, and told her the story, quite annoyed at this point. I peeked in conference room C. Everyone had returned there and was sleeping. Lucky dogs! My contact lenses were so sandpaper-dry I would have to get them out with tweezers. We sat in the downstairs lobby, discouraged, as the House Sup investigated and promised to get back to us. It was then 10:00 p.m. We had to be up at 5:30 a.m. and face another twelve-hour shift and then a drive home afterward, in the snow.

I was beginning to think I should have gone home. But the

temperature outside was dropping, and I pictured myself in a ditch somewhere for a few hours in twelve-degree weather. I thought about Googling nursing jobs in Florida. At that moment, she called.

"Good news!" We needed this. "There's a room that got cancelled in the Cardiac Cath Lab. You can both stay there."

"Okay!" I said, and thanked her profusely. Rose and I gathered our stuff up again. But there was one last problem. I was new and didn't know where the Cath Lab was. Neither did Rose. At the first floor concierge desk was a body. She gave us directions which Rose absorbed but I didn't. I was nearly blind from dry eyes and my mind was fading quickly.

We went through the doors, turned right and went to the end of the hall and turned left, and after the second set of doors turned left again, and through the whatever, and we finally came to the Cath Lab. There we found three night owls with calm smiles, and like cool jazz musicians they eased us over to our room. Those night-shift people were a different, wonderful breed.

Our "room" came equipped with a sink and a TV and a door that closed! And a bathroom right next door! One of the owls brought us a second stretcher and blankets and they both fit comfortably in our room. I texted my husband and boys, safe in their beds at home.

I know this is a First World problem, but this being said, I didn't go camping much! And I really liked and needed my privacy. It's how I re-charged. I was so happy that I could pee and take out my contacts and that our room was like a hotel. We were so tired we didn't even watch the TV. We crashed as soon as we hit the pillows of our stretchers with their side rails up. It was 10:30 p.m., 22:30 hours.

My iPhone gave a "di-doo-di-doo" at 5:30 a.m., 0530 hours, one hour and fifteen minutes before we had to clock in. We slowly awoke, a little sore but rested enough. We gathered our things, wiped down the stretchers, and said goodbye and thanks to those wonderful watchful night people and made our way back up to the fifth floor break room.

There was a single shower in the bathroom there, and M*A*S*H was playing on the TV. We took turns showering. I threw my hair up in a knot and put some makeup on. Breakfast was another swipe of the badge down in the cafeteria. We ate, and I said goodbye to Rose. I texted my husband. He wasn't up yet. I was sure he and the boys were still cozy in bed.

Two of the nurses were late, as expected, but we were glad they made it safely. There was about eight inches of snow on the ground. They said the roads were lousy. Thank God they didn't end up in a ditch. The snow was still falling a little. Some areas had eight inches, some twelve. The second day was always easier at work because I had the same patients and knew them a little. They seemed relieved to see us. They were able to relax and sleep in.

The metal clanking and smells of bacon and pancakes from the food carts filled the hall. But beyond the walls was a cushion of quiet. There is nothing more peaceful than the sound of pure quiet. I stretched and sipped warm coffee and chatted with the other nurses. I was grateful for how it all turned out, but hoped I would never have to spend the night there again. I got shift report and started checking the meds that would be due. No one was awake, so I got out my cell phone and Googled nursing jobs in Florida.

11

The Priest

Black tree limbs reached out toward the dark and light grey clouds on this windy, wintery day. The streets were dry. I was working in the hospital, on the medical-surgical oncology floor. I had taken the job because I loved oncology, but in reality, most oncology treatments were done outpatient at the cancer centers.

It was more of a general medical-surgical floor with patients who had common illnesses and exacerbations of chronic diseases such as congestive heart failure, COPD (chronic obstructive pulmonary disease, or emphysema), abdominal pain, gastrointestinal bleeding, pneumonia, chest pain, and cellulitis (infection of the deeper layers of skin), to name a few. I had wanted to work in the hospital to gain experience, and I did. I gave chemotherapy medications only about every three to six months. I missed the oncology work, but continued to learn, working with adults.

We were a primary care unit, which meant that each nurse had four patients and took care of all of those patients' needs. There was no aide. About a year later, our supervisor obtained approval for one aide for twenty beds. It was set up so that she had no assigned duties except for what we asked of her. Usually an aide handled a range of duties such as taking blood pressure, temperature, pulse (called taking "vital signs"), checking blood sugars, answering call lights, toileting, bathing, things of that nature. At our hospital, an aide had anywhere from eight to twelve patients, which was standard. Our aide's role was different. Her role was not to have assigned duties, but to be a second set of hands for all twenty patients. She was to do tasks when we called and asked for her help. She was busy. When we had patients who needed all of their personal care done for them—feeding, turning every two hours to prevent bedsores in a bedbound patient, anxious patients who pushed the call light every ten minutes (not an exaggeration)—it could be overwhelming.

Hospital work was new for me. I had trouble at first organizing the day and figuring out when to ask for help. After about a year and a half, I developed a system that worked for me. Nurses all developed their own systems. I had a sheet that I referred to as my "brains." It could be folded up and carried in my pocket. The sheet had eight columns. From the top downward was listed the basic information needed to care for each patient: name, room number, date of birth, age, admission date, diagnosis, history, doctors, code status, allergies, bathroom needs, whether the patient could get out of bed by himself or needed help, diabetic needs including room to write down blood sugar results, IV type and place, oxygen needs, telemetry box (heart monitor) number and trends, weight, diet, pertinent labs, wounds, therapies, medication times, plus space for the report from last R.N., orders that haven't been done, tasks, and checkboxes for nursing documentation needed: assessments, care plans, and teaching. On the back I wrote tasks needing to be done, new orders, patient requests and concerns, and significant events of the day. When a patient was discharged, I scratched the column out. When a new patient was admitted, the admitting work was done in the computer and a new column started, along with having all of the new orders done. I am forgetful. This was the system I found that worked for me.

At the beginning of the shift, the nurse had about thirty minutes to gather all of this information from the computer and obtain a report from the previous shift's nurse. Usually that time was when the patients were waking up, from 6:45 a.m. to 7:15 a.m., and calling for their nurses. It was a bit of a conflict of interest. I learned to go with the flow, but it could be tricky. At times we had no aide all day. At times, we had five patients with no aide. We were actually lucky, though. Other hospitals were worse.

One of our biggest responsibilities was safety, all kinds of safety. Hospitals did huge amounts of research, planning, studying, and data collection on safety and especially about preventing falls. Nurses were constantly reminded of this. If a patient fell, in a roundabout way it was considered the nurse's fault. I worked in a hospital that did not reprimand us for falls, but some hospitals did. We didn't want patients to hurt themselves. A fall was a negative mark on a hospital's safety record. It made the hospital look bad, as if safety didn't matter, which was not true. In my opinion, adequate staffing was the best prevention.

Patients, however, sometimes had a different agenda. Their goal was to do what they did before they became sick or injured. Elderly patients especially, when ill, frequently became confused, in denial, and determined. Patients could be impulsive and persistent, and scare the doody out of the nurses. I don't mean the average reasonable, cautious patients, but those who tried to hide how disoriented they were, forgot that their legs were weak, or wait until the last minute to go to the bathroom, then jump up and walk across the room without asking for help. Impulsivity happened frequently in the hospital. So we had bed and chair alarms, and would watch each other's "jumpers," sneaking in with a smile to grab an arm and help them make it to the bathroom in time. From what other nurses told me, in nursing homes patients had the *right* to fall. I found this right a strangely rationalized concept.

Another guideline nurses operated under was that in the state of Missouri, it was the law that medications were to be administered within one hour before or one hour after the time the medication was due. This seemed a wide, reasonable range. But frequently a nurse would become "stuck" with one patient. It could take thirty minutes to an hour to document and crush fifteen different medications, mix them in applesauce, then position the patient in bed so that he wouldn't choke, then beg the weak, elderly confused patient to take the medicine. Add to that cleaning up stool from incontinence that spilled off the disposable pad all over the sheets, an entire occupied bed change, and a patient bath. Then add multiple phone calls and interruptions to the mix and a nurse could easily lose time. One couldn't rush elderly patients. One didn't rush an emotional conversation with a very sick patient.

I stole the time. My biggest difficulties working in the hospital were all of the phone calls and interruptions that left not enough time for my patients. We all helped each other. Most of the time we made it work. I grew to value my precious organizational tool, my "brains," and my fabulous co-workers. We were a great team, a herd of thoroughbreds, walking, trotting, cantering and galloping around the halls to our patients' rooms.

Ours was a Catholic hospital system. Prayers could be heard over the intercom, over the carpeted hallways, in the mornings at 9:00 a.m. There was a sense of caring that the other hospitals didn't have. Caring was actually part of our employee evaluations, which I found pleasantly refreshing. We were "graded" on our level of compassion.

On this particular cold day, the workload was average and manageable. We were adequately staffed. I saw that I had orders to discharge one of my patients already, at 7:00 a.m. I looked to see if all was in order in the patients' computerized chart and saw that I should contact the social worker, which meant she had to polish some details before the patient could leave. The social worker, Naila, came in at 9:00 a.m. I would call her then.

The patient was an eighty-five-year-old priest. Tall and thin, with brown hair cut very short, he wore glasses and had a medium range of depth to his voice. In the report from the night shift nurse I was told he could be a little demanding but in general he was a simple patient. He had pneumonia, and had improved with his treatment of IV antibiotics and cough medicine. He was independent with walking and eating, took his pills without problems and had already showered and dressed himself (at 7:00 a.m.). He didn't use the call light much and when he did, it was for legitimate reasons. He was alert and oriented, which meant not confused. He was in bed 5120, all the way at the end of the hall. All of our rooms were private.

"Good morning, Father," I said squirting my hands with hand-cleanser gel.

"What?" he asked. I waved. "Oh, hello."

"My name is Jessica and I'll be your nurse today," I said loudly as I wrote my name and four-digit number on the whiteboard on the wall. "Can I take your vitals?"

"Sure." He was cordial, and cooperative while I took his blood pressure, temperature and listened to his lungs.

"How do you feel?" I asked.

"Fine. I still have a cough but I feel better."

"You will probably have that cough for a few weeks. You can take the cough medicine for it." He took his medications with no problems. He had a modest breakfast of toast and fruit.

"I saw that the doctor wrote your discharge orders already," I said. He nodded indicating that he knew. "Where do you live?"

"At the St. Raymond's Rectory."

"I saw there was a note, though, from the social worker. I'll see what that's about and let you know, okay? It usually means something else needs to be addressed before you can go. It's probably just about your ride home or something."

"That's fine," he replied. Little did we know. I had some time at this point, so I went about my morning, doing assessments and passing meds. The patient in 5110 called. He wanted pain medication.

"Stef! Can you witness?" I called to one of my co-workers, who was trotting on the way toward a patient's room. I needed to get some morphine. Two nurses were required in order to log in to the medication-dispensing unit, called a Pyxis, to obtain controlled medications. It was a frequent request.

"Sure." She redirected her trot and followed me into the locked med room. I logged into the Pyxis, selected my patient and the drug and placed my index finger on the fingerprint reader. Stef followed, only she used a password to witness instead of a fingerprint.

"You know, I think you are an alien," I joked. Stef had no fingerprints. She was about five feet tall with red hair and most likely had never been a gang member.

"You're onto me," she joked back, grinning. I never did understand the no-fingerprint thing. Years later she would tell me it was from being a "germophobe", and probably from years of vigorous cleaning that started when she was young.

Katy peeked into the med-room. "Can either of you help me boost in seven (meaning room 5107)?" Katy was the charge nurse for the day; she was helping out.

"Sure," I said. We counted the doses of morphine, slammed the drawer shut and logged out. Katy and I walked to the patient's room, gelled our hands, slipped on gloves and met on either side of her patient's bed. Weak patients slid down in their beds all of the time. If the head of the bed is up, the patient slides down. We had to "boost" patients frequently. We set the head of the bed down, to make it flat.

"Put your arms across your chest and lift up your head,"

Katy told the patient, a lady in her eighties. "We're going to pull you up on three. One, two, three." We gripped the half-sized draw-sheet under the patient and pulled her up so that her head was almost at the top of the bed. We straightened out her pillow and covers and put her call light in reach. It was a satisfying feeling. Then my phone rang. "There you go, dear," Katy smiled. "Is there anything else you need?" The lady shook her head and smiled. We put the head of the bed back up, as well as the legs a little, to prevent her sliding down again.

"Thank you," she said.

I answered my phone.

"Can the patient in 5119 have his tray?" It was Gary from dietary, checking to see if the patient had had his blood sugar checked and insulin given yet. If not, he would set the tray on the counter until the nurse completed the task.

"Tell him I'll be in in a minute," I told him. My phone rang again. It was Dr. Matten, the nephrologist.

"Do you have Mr. Nagel in 5109?"

"Yes."

"Good. He is going to need dialysis today. His kidneys are not responding to the treatment. He will need to have a Quinton (temporary dialysis IV line) placed this morning and dialysis this afternoon. I'll put the orders in," she said. I had already started walking to his room, to check.

"Have you told the patient yet?" I asked.

"I just saw him. I think he understands."

"I'll see that he's ready." I looked into the man's room. He was speaking with his wife. I decided to give the patient in 5110 the morphine first, which was a priority, then checked the patient's blood sugar in 5119 so he could eat. About six minutes had passed since I had left the priest's room. The activity was typical.

I saw the rest of my patients, did assessments and passed meds. I readied the patient in 5109 for his procedure and explained the process of dialysis, done on the hospital's fourth floor by the dialysis nurse. When finished I took a little break, eating yogurt and a low-carb muffin in the conference room where Renee and Emily were also attempting to steal breakfast. Renee received a call and had to run. So much for her warm biscuits and gravy. Then I stole a quick pee.

Around 9:20 I phoned Naila. She came to our floor to talk with me about the priest. "The patient in 5120 will need to go to a nursing home so I have to arrange for it," she said.

"Did you know he's a priest? I thought he lived at the rectory," I said, confused.

"I spoke with the rectory this morning," she said. "They have decided to have him move to a nursing home. I'm not sure why. Does he need a lot of personal care?"

"No! That's strange. He is independent! Other than being a little hard of hearing, he doesn't need help with anything. He showered and dressed himself this morning." Nursing homes were for people who needed a lot of personal assistance, or are confused, not for someone like this priest.

"Are you sure they are talking about this patient?" Not that there were a lot of priests in the hospital right then. Maybe she had it mixed up.

"Yes, I am sure," she said. "I'm not really sure why, though. I'll call you when I get more information."

"Have you told the patient yet?" I asked. This would be a blow.

"Not yet. I guess I'm kind of avoiding it," she said. We looked at each other, our expressions changed, and she agreed to break the news.

Outside the open door I sat, feigning computer charting. Naila maintained a professional, positive voice while delivering this life-altering blow. Her words echoed off the walls and tiled floor.

"Hello, Father. I am Naila, the social worker here. I saw

a note in the chart from the weekend social worker to call the place where you live. I called and spoke with the rectory this morning. Apparently, you will be going to a nursing home, not back there. Have you spoken with anyone at the rectory?" She had to speak loudly so that he could hear. I stood up and leaned in for a closer listen.

"No. This is the first I've heard about it," he said, a fragile shake in his voice.

"Maybe you can call them. In the meantime, we have orders from the doctor for your discharge, so I will start looking for nursing homes for you. I will talk to you when I find one, maybe in a few hours, okay?" Naila tried to keep her voice professional, and kind.

"Okay," he said. As Naila moved toward the door, I backed away. I figured this had to be a mistake. I peeked into the room and saw the priest reach for the phone. Maybe there had been a miscommunication.

Naila left and I went in. He asked me how to dial out on the phone. I showed him how to dial "nine" first. He looked at me. There had to be an explanation. He put the phone to his ear. I excused myself.

I returned a little while later. Maybe there had been a misunderstanding. He sat there staring downward. His eighty-five-year-old thin frame was looser now, drawn toward the floor.

"Did you speak to anyone?" I asked, sensing the answer already.

"There was no answer. Forty-one years. I lived and worked there for forty-one years. And Father Michael hasn't even called to tell me or offer me a ride. How do you like that?" he said, his voice weak, as if he didn't even have the energy for anger now. I listened. What could I say? How could I comfort this man now? I had nothing. I felt useless.

Then the words came. "Where God closes a door, he opens

a window," I said. It was all I had. It seemed feeble, silly. He nodded. I stayed to see if he wanted to talk more.

"Would you like me to stay?" I offered. He shook his head.

Naila phoned. They had found a nursing home that would accept his insurance. She informed me that one of the women, Lois, who worked at the rectory would give him a ride to the nursing home. She would be there at 1:00 p.m. It was real.

I began to wonder whether he had done something to deserve this treatment. It really wasn't any of my business. But I had found him to be average, respectful, not overly friendly but not egoistic like some priests I knew. I had no right to ask, so I didn't. I just wondered. Had he mismanaged something? Was he a child molester? Did he anger the wrong priest? I felt it had to be something drastic to cause such treatment, so cold, so harsh. I spoke to my supervisor about it. There was nothing we could do. I felt helpless.

I helped him gather his belongings and put his discharge papers together. Naila had the nursing home approved and over the phone I gave the nurse there a full report with instructions to please be extra kind. The nurse understood. The lady from the rectory called from the lobby to let us know she was there. I wanted to wheel him down myself so I could study her face. I wanted to look into her eyes. I wanted to see righteousness or shame, or some sort of a clue.

He stepped into the wheelchair with his single bag of belongings. "I can't even go back and get my things. I got a hold of Lois, the secretary who is giving me a ride, on the phone. She says they are having my things sent over."

"I'm so sorry, Father," I said. The tops of my ears burned. What kind of people were these?

"Forty-one years." He just shook his head. He was not fully present.

As I wheeled him down the long hall, I tried to be positive

for him. I spoke loudly. "I've heard really nice things about Delmun Gardens, the place you are going to live."

"Really?" He perked up a little.

"We have patients from there in the hospital here all the time. The residents and their families seem to really like it there."

As I pushed the wheelchair hoping his new thoughts would bring some comfort, another priest came bounding swiftly toward us. I recognized him. He visited our hospital occasionally. He was a short thin man in his late 60s with a crisp white full head of hair, wearing a full black suit and white collar.

He approached Father in a rush and tumbled over him with a prayer. I offered to pull the wheelchair aside but he declined and did his visit right in the middle of the hallway. "In the name of the Father, the Son—" He made the Sign of the Cross. Father could not hear him. The priest didn't speak loudly enough. He quickly finished his babble, patted Father on the shoulder, turned and walked back toward the elevator. Father sat in his wheelchair. His eyes held on to the brisk black frame of the visiting priest until he disappeared around the corner at the end of the hall. He seemed to have needed this encounter desperately, but couldn't hear it, nor fit a word in edgewise. Clearly a disappointment.

Lois was waiting downstairs so I pushed the wheelchair swiftly down the wide, carpeted hall. I was surprised to see the visiting priest still there, waiting for the elevator. As we entered, he went first as I backed Father's wheelchair in, so he could face the doors. The visiting priest stood at the back next to me.

"These old geezers, half the time they can't hear anything," he began, as if telling me a secret. "When I was in seminary, we had a professor that couldn't hear so we'd play tricks on him. We would all speak really quietly so he had to ask 'What?' during class, then we'd all speak loudly at once to shock the old guy!" He giggled and elbowed my arm like a middle-school boy bragging about a prank.

I turned to him, allowing my face to express the truth: pure disgust. I didn't explain. There was no reason for such disrespect. Thank goodness my patient had not heard. The elevator opened and I glared as the visiting priest took off running.

By the front doors of the hospital, Lois stood there with the car door open. I tried to read her. I couldn't simply ask what was going on. The priest asked her why Father Michael hadn't given him a ride. She acted as if he had annoyed her, and told him Father Michael was busy.

He grabbed his coat to wrap himself as a cold wind suddenly brushed through the circular driveway in front of the hospital. Like prickly ice it slapped our unprotected faces.

"Let's get in the car," she said impatiently. She stood holding the car door, shaking her head. She gave me a half smile. "Let's get a move on." He wasn't seated yet when she walked around to the driver's side and seated herself.

"Goodbye, Father," I said, my hand on his shoulder. He nodded and then they were gone.

I could speculate that he had done really bad things. I could speculate that the church was very militaristic, rearranging men like chess pieces on a board. But I would think that a Sergeant or Major would say goodbye or at least acknowledge the comings and goings of men. Or someone would. I heard that the church did things like that. None of this was comforting. I'll never know why.

Perhaps I shouldn't know. What I guess I was meant to know was that an eighty-five-year-old man who had devoted his life to the service of the church was told he could no longer live there. And he was full of sadness. Maybe I'm only meant to know how to offer kindness during terrible times no matter what the story, or at least let the words pass through me.

12

Choices

Years ago, I went to high school for the first two years in St Louis, and then the last two years in Maryland. Not many teachers made an impression with the exception of one, Mrs. Hall, who taught freshman English. Not because I liked the subject or that her class was in mid-morning when I started to wake up each day, but because of her. She had a calm, relaxed, go-with-the-flow nature. She was short, plain-looking and had short brown hair.

We were teenagers and full of moods, hormones, gossip, social pressure and intense intellectual challenges. She had us sit in a circle in class most of the time to encourage conversation. She respected us and treated us like people. She was the teacher that the kids went to when they had trouble or needed help. She had a way of calling foul when we were out of line yet still treating us as if we were special, accepted, part of "her group." She was beloved. But I moved on, and eventually moved to the state of Maryland, and forgot.

* * *

I was working in the hospital. I had a patient who was very sick. She had cancer in its advanced stages and her husband wanted everything done to save her. She needed blood transfusions, albumin, IV antibiotics and fluids. She had terrible skin breakdown from the cancer that oozed and required frequent care which was extremely painful, despite the IV pain medicine. Her skin was fire-engine red and raw.

Her poor body was swollen to almost twice its size, full of fluid from her failing kidneys. Her face was moon-shaped. Her arms were taut from the swelling, with skin pale pink and thin. We elevated them on pillows. She was suffering, confused, unaware and had a very poor prognosis. There were no more cancer treatment options.

The wound nurse specialist, Maureen, was also involved, to help find the best way to care for her wounds. She came to see my patient. Maureen called the patient's husband "Coach."

"Why do you call him 'Coach'?" I asked after she completed her assessment. I figured she knew him.

"He was our coach for my old high-school football team. I was a cheerleader. Everyone liked Coach. That was only, like, forty years ago! God, that's a crazy thought!" We laughed. She was tall and thin with brown straight hair cut in a face frame, and an excellent nurse. She wore those years well.

"You mean like ten years, right?" I teased.

"Yeah, that's it! Ha! Well, Coach was nails. He was tough on the guys, but they needed it. When he spoke, you were expected to listen. We had a great team! Now that I'm a grownup, I can see that he's strict but really an old softy. Seeing him makes it feel like it was just yesterday." She looked at the wall, then smiled and smacked me with her folder and went back to work. "See ya."

"See ya."

"Coach" was about six feet five inches tall and solid. He had a bit of a southern drawl, much like Dr. Phil the psychologist who has a show on TV, with a soft, raspy voice, probably from years of screaming in the great outdoors to a bunch of teenage boys full of energy. Although I was not into sports and had not been around his type much, I could tell he had wisdom. His daughter was with him, dressed like an athlete, wearing jogging pants and a jacket and sneakers. They talked about the details of the strategy of her son's technique in soccer. He talked to her about conditioning and the ball and movements, those sporty things I pretty much know nothing about. I had tried all kinds of sports with my boys: baseball, soccer, basketball, even Tae Kwon Do. They didn't like sports and would have nothing to do with them. They were into Scouts and band, science and art. Our middle son did compete in fencing, if that counts. I do yoga and the treadmill. That's the extent of our athletics. And my husband works. A lot. That's his sport.

Although I didn't really understand this type of person, he struck me as an honorable soul. I admired him. I saw years of him helping kids, a family man. But now, mostly what I saw was hope. The worst kind: false hope.

I saw it a lot in my profession. We hear what we want to hear and see what we want to see when it comes to our loved ones. We can't imagine one who laughed and lived and worked and raised children and loved us so consistently might not exist anymore. We can't imagine not helping them, not doing everything we could. I know I would.

There's an old story that I'm reminded of that goes like this: If you toss a frog into boiling water, he'll jump right out. Put him in tepid water and slowly turn up the heat and he will stay in, slowly cooking to his demise.

That was what I seemed to walk into that day. It probably happened gradually, over days or weeks—her decline. By that afternoon I had cleaned her skin maybe eight times. She screamed in pain each time. I gave her morphine, dilaudid, topical lidocaine, and was very gentle, but nothing seemed to work. I had to close her door each time. It seemed more like a torture chamber than a hospital, dark and medieval. I knew the other patients had heard. Not all cancers end like this. I was in her room constantly. My other patients were neglected. I had to ask for help, frequently. It felt like we were forcing her to live when her poor body wanted to die.

She wouldn't eat at this point. I don't think she could have. Coach would encourage her to no avail. He would sit by her, hold her hand, and keep faith. I wasn't sure what the doctors had said to him or if they had spoken to him about her code status. I called the primary-care doctor but he had not returned my call yet and several hours had gone by. I didn't see anything in his notes. The oncologist had painted a clear, bleak picture in her note in the patient's chart and had signed off of her case, which was the norm, leaving her care to her primary doctor, who would be responsible from then on. The oncologists would still visit, unofficially, while patients were in the hospital. It seemed that there was a break in communication, though, with Coach. He didn't seem to understand what was going on, and continued to try to feed her. I finally spoke to the primary doctor later that day. He gave approval to discuss the code status with Coach and to order whatever Coach decided. I told the charge nurse and went forward with the most difficult discussion.

"Mr. Hall, can I speak with you a minute?"

He was in a daze, exhausted. He had switched roles and become her cheerleader. He sat on the couch on the other side of her hospital room—the hospital had all private rooms—and I sat in the chair. Mrs. Hall slept.

"I'm not sure if the doctors have discussed this with you. I think they may have, but I wanted to ask you, have you thought about what she would want if her heart would stop beating or if she would stop breathing?"

"We have an advance directive. She doesn't want to be on a breathing machine. But she's breathing fine."

It was as I had thought. He didn't really understand how it worked. The choices could be very confusing. Sometimes we don't realize what they are. The whole hospital experience can be confusing. He was doing his best, though, acting as her strength. But his wife was going to die from this.

"There's another thing we need to talk about. It's called code status. Right now, because she has full code status, if her heart would stop we would fully resuscitate her. We would push hard on her chest for chest compressions, possibly breaking her ribs. If she stopped breathing, we would put a tube into her throat and attach her to an ambu bag, then possibly a ventilator at least temporarily to make her breathe, give her all kinds of medications to keep her alive. Is this what she would want?"

He looked at me strangely.

"But we have a living will."

"So you have power of attorney and her wishes, that's good. And we would take her off of the ventilator later if that's what it says to do. But while she is here, we need to clarify what she would want us to do if anything would happen now. All patients have the option of which care they would want if the extreme happens. If people are otherwise healthy, they would usually choose 'full code' and we would do everything to save them should the worst happen. Pretty much everyone who is admitted has full code status unless it is changed by the hospitalist doctor or primary-care doctor.

"But when a person is ill and there will probably not be a chance of recovery, they can choose to select only some of the nine or so choices, such as no intubation—a breathing tube in her trachea—no CPR, no defibrillator, which is a 'partial code' or 'partial DNR' status.

"If you want nothing to be done if her heart stops or she stops breathing, you would choose a do-not-resuscitate code status, or DNR. We could still continue all of the rest of her care.

"But when someone is very ill, many people may choose to be a DNR and withdraw treatment and shift the focus from curing the person to making them comfortable, which is hospice. You can choose anything you believe she would want. Does that make sense?"

He seemed to have not heard this before, or maybe he hadn't wanted to. He seemed to shift. And then this big, strong, wise, confident man wept.

He began to realize the unthinkable. I sat with him, I'm not sure for how long. Time stands still in moments like this.

"Would you like me to stay?" I asked. He shook his head.

A while later, he pressed the call light and when I went in told me of his decision. We called the doctor and received the order to change her code status to a DNR. He decided to withdraw all treatment. I was off the next day but heard she died in less than twenty-four hours. She was finally at peace.

About a year later, a very long time it seemed, I saw Coach again in the hall on our floor. I was surprised.

"Hi, Coach!" I said. He seemed to be the same. Back straight, a formal handshake.

"What are you doing here?" Maybe there was another sick family member.

"I just wanted to come by and see you and Maureen, to say thanks," he said.

Wow, I hadn't expected that.

"I was up at her high school and thought I'd swing by."

"How sweet! Thank you! What high school? I didn't realize she taught too." I had been so busy with her intense care needs when she was my patient I hadn't learned anything about her.

"She taught English at Kennedy South," he replied. Then it hit me like a ton of bricks. She was Mrs. Hall. My beloved English teacher! I hadn't thought of her name in years. I hadn't put the two together. When it had happened the year before, I had not recognized her. I felt so stupid.

"Mr. Hall, I am just realizing, I didn't know she taught there. That was my high school! I had her freshman year! I didn't

Jessica Patton, R.N.

recognize her or realize when I took care of her. I'm so sorry.
I feel so silly! She was so wonderful. We all loved her. I know
that's how you remember her, not your horrible time here!" I
was falling all over my words, more so because of my shock
and grief. How she suffered at the end. How nasty cancer is.

"It took me a long time before I could come back to thank
you," he said.

"I can't imagine," I stammered. "But it's good to see you.
Thank you for coming by! I can't believe it was her. You were
so strong for her; I admired that." I was still stunned. "Would
you like me to see if Maureen's here?" I asked.

"If you would," he said. I searched her office, which was on
the same floor, but no Maureen. I called her phone and checked
with my boss. She was at another hospital in a meeting.

I came back to find him sitting there, patiently waiting.
Alert, hands on his knees, face flat, but with a sadness. I think
he was remembering. I couldn't help but think that if I could
remember her wonderfulness, I'm sure he could look past this
place, too.

"She's not here. Would you like me to tell her you came
by?"

"Would you? I may stop by next week. I wanted to thank
her, too."

"Okay, Coach, I will. And Coach," I interjected, feeling a
lump in my throat, "she was wonderful. Everyone loved her."

He shook my fumbling hand. I wanted to hug him, but didn't
think he was the hugging type. And he left. It had taken him a
year to come back. What a courageous and wonderful man. I
wish I'd known him better.

And I thought about Mrs. Hall. Her smile, her kindness,
her no-B.S. way of handling us. Her calmness. Her love of the
language. Her wisdom. Her way of not letting things get to her.
I soaked her in. And cursed death and felt her life.

13

Ethan

E than was in the outfield, playing softball for his physical-education class as he had done dozens of times before. It was only eighty degrees, a sunny day in May. He sized up the hitter, looked around at a runner on base and at the other outfielders, and thought about his last few days of high school. He was a senior. He would miss this place, but was ready to move on. The batter swung and missed. The sunlight got brighter for Ethan, and then it faded. As if playing a game of trust, he felt his body leaning back, but didn't feel the ground.

A coach yelled out, "It's Ethan Brock!" Like a well-oiled machine, as if rehearsed, kids came running. The coach listened for breathing; there was none. He felt Ethan's neck. The pulse was barley palpable and erratic.

"Get help, get the AED!!" he screamed. An AED is a box-like medical device programmed to detect heart rates through two sticky pads placed on the bare chest and deliver a shock to reset the heart if needed. A second coach appeared out of nowhere. He was supposed to be at a golf tournament that day but for some reason hadn't gone. Only the coaches, and of course the nurse, were required to be trained in CPR at the school.

Several years ago, another student had collapsed and died at this school while at football practice. Ethan had turned blue. This had happened to him before. Four months before in January, Ethan had collapsed in gym class but had regained consciousness right away. Hence, the well-oiled machine of preparedness. They had sent him to the hospital and ran all the tests. They had even sent him home with a heart monitor he had to wear for six weeks. Everything was negative. But it was happening again.

This time they were prepared. The coach, who never carried his cellphone to the field, just happened to have it that day. He phoned 911 and began describing Ethan's fall, his blue color, and said they were starting CPR. The second coach leaned over and pinched off Ethan's nose, tilted his head back, and placed his mouth over Ethan's mouth. He gave two breaths. He felt for the proper placement on Ethan's chest, put one hand on top of the other, straightened his arms and pushed. 1...2...3...4...5...6...7...8...9...10. All the way to 30, then two more breaths, then 1...2...3...4...5...6...7...8...9...10, to 30 again.

The nurse and a third coach, who had come in only to do paperwork that day, arrived. They placed the two AED pads on his chest. "ANALYZING RHYTHM," its digital voice said. That was the sign to stop chest compressions so the AED could evaluate the heart activity. "SHOCKABLE RHYTHM, PLEASE STAND CLEAR."

They stood back a little from Ethan's body so they would not also receive the shock. "BEEEEEEEP!" "ZZZZZTT." Ethan's fragile chest lifted slightly, then relaxed. Everyone was silent except the AED.

"RESUME CPR." The second coach gave Ethan two more breaths, and began again. 1...2...3...4..., to 15 this time, as the nurse stepped in for two-person CPR. After two more rounds, the AED spoke.

"ANALYZING RHYTHM." It paused. "SHOCKABLE RHYTHM, PLEASE STAND CLEAR." The coach and nurse stood back. "BEEEEEEP!" "ZZZZZTTT." Ethan's chest rose with the shock, and then fell. "RESUME CPR." The coach and nurse continued CPR.

Ethan's lips were blue. His skin was white. His friends were afraid. They expected him to wake up and say, "Ha! Just kidding!" but he did not move. The coaches and nurse looked at each other, then toward the parking lot. *Where was that ambulance?* they thought, while pushing on Ethan's lifeless sternum. It had been only about five minutes, possibly more, but it seemed an eternity.

The ambulance arrived and the paramedics were calm and cool. Then they saw Ethan, and their adrenalin and training kicked in. Ethan's young, limp body being pushed on by adults in order to keep his heart going was enough to make anyone cry out inside, *Come on, start beating!*

One paramedic resumed chest compressions where the nurse had left off. The other grabbed oxygen connected to an ambu bag: a rubber, balloon-like bag attached to a facemask that is squeezed to provide breaths to the patient. He pushed much-needed oxygen into Ethan's lungs. Coach quickly told them what had happened. They rolled Ethan onto a stretcher and into the ambulance. Then, like lightning, with sirens and lights flashing, they were gone.

The coaches, nurse, teachers, and students were left standing on the field. Coming down from their adrenaline rush, they stood and watched and breathed. The air was still. What had just happened? What would happen now?

The coaches and staff then took charge, arms around the students and each other. The leaders and their followers went back inside the high school.

In the next town over, Ed, a local business owner and Ethan's father, was sitting at a stoplight, his heart pounding so hard the liquid spilled out through his eyes and ran down his face. He was trying to will the light to turn green, but it hadn't worked so far. He was on his cellphone to his ex-wife, Ethan's mother Jennifer, or Jen, as I called her. He told her what he knew.

"I don't know if he is alive or not. All they said was that it is very serious. I'm on my way to the hospital, St. Catherine."

"What happened? Is it his heart?" Jen asked.

"It happened at school. I don't know. That's all I know," he said. "I'll see you there."

It so happened that Jen was in nursing school at the time, studying be an R.N. In her forties, Jen was small, with a dazzling smile and an impossibly delicate strength. She had a degree in psychology but had never worked in the field because she wanted to be a stay-at-home mom, and did that for many years. She homeschooled her older kids for a few of those years and was always carting them around to activities and meetings with the homeschooling co-op. She had six children. Five were girls ranging from three years old to twenty. Ethan was eighteen, her second child and only son. Jen had always been fascinated with the human body and how it functioned, and wanted to make her own income. She was at the end of her second semester in nursing school and had two more to go.

It's very serious. It's very serious. She kept replaying the phrase over and over in her head: "*It's very serious.*" The words echoed in her mind as she was turning her car around to leave her daughters' school where she had been meeting with a teacher. It seemed she was helpless to manipulate time and space to be with her only son. Her legs moved much too slowly, her hand grabbed for the keys for what seemed like forever in the black hole that was her purse. She climbed into the van and had to re-think each action to start the ignition and drive the vehicle out of the parking lot and onto the road. She had to drive the speed limit so when she made it onto the highway, she set the cruise control. She had about thirty miles to go.

She called her mother, her husband, and some of her friends while she drove, and prayed for help to prepare for whatever she would find. Talking made it more real to her; it was too much to comprehend. She called a friend from her church to spread the word. She put it in God's hands and asked for strength and trust.

I was working at St. Catherine Hospital that day when I received her call.

"Are you working?" Jen said, her voice just a little shaky. We had been good friends for more than thirty years.

"Yes. How are you?" I couldn't really tell how anxious she was, but I did notice a quiver in her voice. Jen had a way of making everything seem calm and normal, all of the time.

"Ethan collapsed on the field at school again. The coaches had to do CPR this time! He's on his way to the E.R. there at St. Catherine." She was trying to keep from crying, I could tell.

I let out an audible gasp. "Oh, Jen! Is he okay?"

"All I know is that they did CPR and had to shock him twice. They said it's very serious!"

"I'll go down to the E.R. and check in a few minutes. Are you close?"

"I'll be there in a few minutes."

"I'll say some prayers. I'll meet you down there."

"Okay."

"Love you, Jen."

"Love you, too."

I tried to place myself in her shoes. How could someone begin to contemplate the possible loss of a child? I couldn't imagine it. I think we're equipped with denial so as not to have our minds and hearts collapse during these significant moments.

I finished passing meds to my patients. It was morning. I told the charge nurse what was happening and she agreed to keep an eye on my patients. We, the nurses, carried phones called Ascoms wherever we went. The charge nurse could reach me if necessary. I took the elevator from our fifth floor down to the first floor and the E.R., which was not busy that day; not very many patients were there. I prepared myself, making my back straight, preparing my arms to hold my grief-stricken friend if need be.

Jen finally arrived, parked and saw an ambulance and a paramedic near the entrance. *The paramedic must know,* she thought. The hospital was only twelve minutes from the high school. Her breathing was heavy. Her heart resembled a basketball dribbling inside her chest as her body took over, moving her shaky legs toward the only ambulance there. *This could be the worst news of a lifetime,* she thought. *"It's very serious"* still rang in her head. She ran toward him.

"Did you come from Eureka High School? My son Ethan was brought here. Was it you who brought him?" Jen asked, her voice raised and shrill.

"Are you a relative?" the paramedic asked.

"Yes, his mother. Is he alive?"

"Yes, ma'am. He's inside. They're working on him now."

"Thank you!" This was a start! She could at least breathe. She jogged into the E.R. The triage nurse knew who she was when she entered. Jen's green eyes were wide with adrenalin and urgency. The nurse showed Jen where Ethan was. Ed and his fiancée were there signing papers; Ed covered Ethan on his health insurance plan. Jen's mother was on her way.

St. Catherine was a small but new hospital, with state-of-the-art equipment and experienced doctors and staff. Usually trauma patients went to the bigger hospitals around town. This was not trauma, though, it was something else.

I went down through the E.R. and saw a security guard that I knew. I told him what was happening and that Jen was a close friend. He showed me to Ethan's room. It was a single-bed room, brightly lit and filled with equipment. My neighbor Emily was Ethan's nurse, but so were most of the rest of the E.R. nurses right then, all helping however they could. About fifteen people—doctors, nurses, phlebotomists, respiratory therapists, pharmacists, security guards, X-ray techs, other staff, and Jen—were lining Ethan's room as the nurses worked on him.

Jen watched with no expression as he lay motionless. A tube in his mouth went into his trachea, attached to a ventilator or breathing machine. Ed was outside of the room. The E.R. doctor and the intensivist (ICU) doctor were looking at numbers and monitors, examining Ethan and giving orders verbally. Ethan's heart had started beating on its own. The rhythmic green line of the heart monitor above his bed showed a steady *blip, blip, blip,* which was encouraging, but he was not stabilized yet.

My eyes met Jen's and I mouthed a whisper to her from across the crowded room, "Hey." She was standing to the side of Ethan's bed, toward the head.

"Hey," she mouthed in return, and smiled, then returned her gaze to him.

To Jen's surprise, it was our hospital's policy to allow the family to stay in Ethan's E.R. room as long as she was able to handle it emotionally, and not in the way of the staff while they were working. She watched as the doctor placed a central IV line, a larger IV tube about six inches long, into the large vein at the base of Ethan's neck. A larger IV like this can handle multiple medications and was not in danger of dislodging or weakening as can smaller single IVs in the hands or arms.

"Do you think he's in pain?" Jen asked one of the nurses.

"No. We've given him medicine to sedate him. He will be unconscious for a while," the nurse said.

"Why are his arms twitching?" Jen asked.

"Sometimes when the brain doesn't receive enough oxygen, the nerves can spasm and there can be twitching like that," the nurse said. Jen was concerned. When they were able to talk, she would have to ask the doctors about this.

The nurses gave him more medications. They cleared the room of people. Jen cringed as Emily explained that they were inserting a nasogastric tube from his nose into his stomach to drain it and keep stomach acid from entering his lungs while he was sedated. They would also insert a Foley catheter tube into his bladder. Jen knew what these tubes were, having inserted them in patients in her clinical rotations at the hospital. Jen, her parents, Ed, his fiancée and I all moved into a waiting room nearby. I greeted them and turned to Jen and hugged her. Her eyes were wet, and a tissue was affixed to her fist.

"They say they don't know how long his brain went without oxygen, and he's doing this twitching thing with his arms," she said. "They're calling a neurologist and a cardiologist to see him. They're going to transfer him to the ICU in a little while."

"Jen, I'm so glad he's alive! I wasn't sure what I would find when I came down here!"

"I didn't know for the entire way over here from St. Charles, thirty miles!"

"What a nightmare."

Jen took a deep breath. We sat down.

"So, does being in nursing school help or hinder?" I asked.

"It kind of helps. I understand things better. I'm flipping back and forth from feeling like a nurse to feeling like a mom. The nurse role is easier."

We exchanged knowing glances. I could see that. The nurse role is like putting on your best face and leaving your troubles at the door. It's work. The mom role is helpless, silently begging each and every person caring for your son to *Please be careful, please do your best, he is extremely precious to me!* I knew our staff, though. I knew how gentle, knowledgeable, and caring they were. He was in the right place.

I cringed sympathetically and went with the idea of her "nurse role." "I guess that's a good thing!" I said. A doctor approached, so I chose a seat by Jen's mom. Jen and Ed listened astutely to his explanation of the course of action. A few friends trickled in through the E.R. doors along with more family and some staff from the high school. Jen went over to speak with them, just outside of Ethan's room. A few men were standing there. It seemed like they were probably the coaches from Ethan's school.

When Jen was finished, she came back to the waiting room. "The doctor says they don't know how long his brain went without oxygen when his heart stopped." The body can only go on for minutes without blood and oxygen.

"They don't know what caused it or what damage has been done, especially to his brain. Apparently he's not necessarily okay yet. Right now they need to focus on preserving his brain. He said the more recent studies show that the best course of action to preserve brain function is to cool the body for twenty-four hours under a cooling blanket. He said that when the heart stops like this it is usually either neurological, or heart-related. They need to do more tests, but they need to do the cooling blanket now." She was trying to absorb this information as she explained it to us. Her family digested the news. "The thing is," Jen was reluctant to explain, "apparently it takes twelve hours to cool his body down, then twenty-four hours at a target temperature of thirty-three degrees Celsius (91.4 degrees Fahrenheit), then twelve hours to warm him back up. Two days." It seemed a lifetime. Two days. *"What damage had been done."* The words echoed in her mind. The doctors didn't know *what damage had been done.*

Back in Ethan's room, Emily moved monitors and applied stickers to his chest to rearrange the leads for a portable heart monitor, preparing to move him to the ICU. Emily and several other nurses were still working on Ethan. She looked at me, and looked at Jen, and with compassion, looked at Ethan, then back at Jen. In her busyness, it was her way of expressing the thought, *I can't imagine what you're going through; we will take good care of your son.*

A moment of no words passed as Jen struggled to keep

her cool. She silently vowed to be strong for him. Her mind wandered back to moments in time sealed with his sweetness: As a little blond toddler with big brown eyes he had wanted to sing a special song to her. He had a red toy microphone with a button that made the sound of applause when pushed. He called his mom to sit on the couch so he could sing a special "ABC's of you" song to her.

She could picture the rich wood flooring beneath his tiny little feet in the big A-frame great room of their house in the woods. He had held so tightly to the microphone, trembling with determination, singing straight from his heart, wearing nothing but a diaper and a blue cape. When he finished he pushed the applause button, and full of pride said, "Clap, Mommy, clap!" She clapped heartily and laughed and welcomed him into her arms with hugs and kisses.

Now he was tall with broad shoulders and a soft-spoken deep voice. He was almost an adult, with a girlfriend and college plans. She was proud of the person he had become. He should be beginning his own life. I believe that a mother sees her child in a unique, timeless way: a baby, a toddler, a school-aged child, and a teenager—she sees them all as one.

They had stabilized him enough to move him to the ICU. I noticed on the way to the elevator that his arms kept rising in a "posturing" position, curved and raised up slightly above his hips. It was a repeated reminder of a possible sign of brain damage, the doctor had warned. He was in a chemically induced coma and on a ventilator.

A team of protective nurses and the intensivist doctor ascended with Ethan and his machines up the elevator to the third floor, which would be his new home for a while. Jen, Ed and a few family members took the next elevator. Jen asked her husband, who had been on standby for instructions at home, to coordinate her younger girls' needs with Jen's mother and bring to the hospital Jen's nursing textbooks, phone charger, some clothes, and a toothbrush so she could study while camping out in Ethan's private hospital room. She didn't want the younger girls to see Ethan just yet. She would stay there for the duration. We all had to wait for two days. I went back to work on the fifth floor. It was difficult to switch back to being a nurse that day.

Down in the ICU, the nurses covered Ethan with the cooling blanket and started his preservation. The countdown had begun. I finished my shift and would be off for a few days. A Facebook post on Jen's wall asked for prayers for Ethan. I "Liked'" it. I checked on Jen and Ethan before I left.

"How is he?" I asked.

"He's cooling down." The monitor read 35 degrees; the target was 33. "He still does that posturing thing with his arms every so often. It's so unnerving. I can't believe we won't know for two days whether I'll get my Ethan back or not. What if he has brain damage? What if he can't function? His whole life could change. He could need to be fed and have to wear a diaper." She stopped. She tried not to tear up again. I touched her forearm, knowing she might be correct.

"Or he could be just fine."

"Yes, he could be just fine," I agreed.

"I know," she said. "I just can't imagine him that way. I just have to believe he's going to be okay."

"I saw your Facebook post, so you have about a million people praying for him! The odds are in your favor," I said. She smiled and agreed. But in my mind, it could have gone either way.

"Talk about a lesson in patience," she groaned. I agreed. I noticed there were nursing textbooks lying around, open, with papers on top of and next to them.

"Looking things up, are we?" I said. Nurses and nursing students know just enough to be dangerous sometimes. We know the simple medical ideas, but they can become very complex and take a lot more digging to understand. It can be a good way of learning, though. But with Ethan, we didn't have a diagnosis yet. The doctors and nurses were only supporting him and reacting to what had happened. His was not a simple or typical problem.

"As if this weren't enough, I have a nursing final in three days!"

"I think your instructor would give you an extension, don't you? Under the circumstances?" I said, but it was pointless. I would have never been able to focus during a time like that, but that was me. I knew Jen. She had more energy than God ever intended to give one person, and the brainpower to match. She looked at me with a grin. "I've been praying and I think God knows what I want to happen. I can't just sit here and worry. It gives me something to do!"

"I can see that. You're going to make a great nurse." We talked a little more and said our goodbyes. It had been a long day.

The next morning, Jen and I shared texts:

Good morning, u up?

Yep, been up since 6

Did u sleep ok?

Not too bad, strange though, all the noises

Yeah, the hosp is noisy. Is he ok?

Yeah, 33 deg, just waiting

Can I buy u breakfast?

Not too hungry but sure

K, be by in a bit ;)

K ;)

Jen appeared sleepy when I arrived mid-morning. Ed and his fiancée and Ethan's grandparents were there keeping watch. Ethan's sisters were at home with Jen's husband. We went downstairs to the cafeteria. It was carpeted in the seating area and smelled of bacon and muffins. I ate a muffin and we shared some fresh fruit. Jen, of course, was worrying about everyone else: the kids, her husband, her mom, and the nurses. It kept her busy. That was a good thing, keeping busy. In retrospect, she was radiating strength.

"Have you ever heard of 'Healing Touch'?" I asked her.

"I've heard of it, but refresh my memory," Jen said.

"It's used sometimes with cancer patients but is really for anyone. It's a theory that our human touch has an energy that has a healthy effect on the body, heart, mind and spirit. Practitioners are trained to focus intentional supportive energy using their hands, by touching and holding the hands just above the body. We have a Healing Touch program here and two of my friends who are nurses are practitioners of it."

"I've heard of it. It sounds good."

"It's an informal program. It's free. Would you be interested in having them come do a session for Ethan? I could call them if you'd like. I think they are here today."

"It sounds nice. Every little bit helps," she said.

"I'll give them a call," I said. "How are the girls taking it?"

"Allison and Audrey don't really understand, they're so little, but I think they sense how serious it is. Emma and Olivia are upset but praying hard. They'll be up later. Hannah is coming up from college today. She wants to be here with him." We talked about her girls and my three boys and anything to pass the time.

A little while later, I made some calls and set up the Healing Touch session. The rest of the family wouldn't be there until later. That afternoon, the nurses Peggy and Nicklette came into Ethan's room with a CD player, greeted Jen and me, and dimmed the lights. All the doctors had seen Ethan and would make no more changes to his care. It was now a waiting game. Peggy put a "do-not-disturb" sign on the door. Jen and I sat on the couch in his room facing the foot of his bed. They scooted the six IV pumps mounted on a pole aside just a little bit. Faint, calming flute music began playing in the background. The sound of the ventilator breathing in, *siiiip,* then out, *whoooosh,* over and over was a reminder amidst the peace.

Jen sat upright, alert, her back stiff. Her face was expressionless; her resolve was a mixture of anxiety and strength. Slowly, with focused energy, Peggy and Nicklette moved the silvery grey cooling blanket down his body a little, and held out their hands to gently touch Ethan's shoulders, arms, chest, legs, neck and head. Jen and I silently watched. Later, when I asked, Jen told me that she had her own vision that she played over and over in her mind during the session: Ethan waking up and saying, "Mom." She refused to give in to the alternative. We thanked the nurses for the Healing Touch session. We all hugged and I left and went home.

Jen studied. She visited with friends and family. She thrived on all of the company and support. Her husband, older girls and daughter from college, Hannah, came. Hannah stayed at the hospital that night. Someone from administration at Ethan's school visited. Finally around 11:00 p.m., exhausted, she fell asleep.

The next morning, seeing my boys off to school, I went back to sleep until about 9:30. The target time for removing the blanket and seeing him wake up was 11:00 a.m. At this point, Ed, Jen and Ethan's sisters had had so much support, so many visitors and so many good thoughts and prayers, that they managed to keep going despite their exhaustion. Hannah wore a T-shirt with the word HOPE across the chest. Ethan's girlfriend sat by his side.

Jen, Ed and the rest of the family, except for the little girls, stared at his expressionless face, dotted with stubble. Soon they would know. The monitor read 36.9 degrees Celsius. The new target was 37 degrees. They observed the blue corrugated ventilator tube connected to a smaller white one that went down his throat, a central IV line in his neck with about seven tubes feeding into it, patches for the cardiac monitor peeking out from under the ugly brown-and-green hospital gown, the grey cooling blanket. Hannah took a few photos to show him later.

The monitor on the blanket read 37 degrees. The nurse removed the cooling blanket from his body. The intensivist doctor had written orders and was standing by. The nurses began weaning Ethan off of the coma-inducing drugs. They turned off the ventilator and let him take practice breaths on his own. He breathed in and out. They removed the tube from his throat. He was breathing on his own but still unconscious. Jen prepared herself for whatever would be. *Come on, baby! You can do it!* she thought.

No one knew what his condition would be when he woke up. He might be in a persistent vegetative state where the brain no longer perceives and expresses: a virtual vegetable. He might never regain consciousness. Or he might be the Ethan everyone knew: a son, a grandson, a brother, a boyfriend, and a friend.

His parents, older sisters, girlfriend, and grandparents surrounded him. *What damage had been done*? Jen thought. She was about to find out. His arms rose again in a curved, tense fashion and then went back down. Jen, standing by the head of his bed, grabbed his left hand. The silence was deafening. They waited.

Ethan opened his eyes. Jen's heart felt like a basketball again. Ethan tried to focus. He focused on Jen, who was about to burst. She smiled at him.

He opened his mouth as I happened to come to his door to witness his first word. In a whisper, he said "Mom?" Her wish had come true! He spoke, he recognized her! He looked around the room, groggy and clueless as to what had happened.

His dad did a happy dance and screamed, "Yeah!" I sighed,

smiling, a happy pressure in my throat. The nurse cheered. The doctor in the doorway stepped back and smiled.

Everyone breathed breaths they had held for days. They felt giddy and light. His family gently eased him into understanding what had happened. Jen let her tears flow. She made sure he wasn't overwhelmed by the lights, sounds, and people. She waited for him to speak.

"Hannah, why did you come home from college?" Ethan said to his sister, in a scratchy voice. Everyone laughed.

"Your heart stopped beating. They had to do CPR on you! You had to be shocked twice. You have been in a medically-induced coma for two days under a cooling blanket to preserve your brain function." He tried to absorb all of the information.

"You drove all the way from Southwest Missouri State to see *me*?"

"Ethan, you almost died!" It was becoming clearer to him. "You're my baby brother; of course I'm going to come up. We thought we might lose you!" She held onto his arm and smiled at him. He looked around the room and began to understand what all of the people were doing there.

"But Mom, what about school, and graduation!? I have finals!" This was his biggest concern. He was a senior, in the Missouri A+ Program, and if he followed certain rules, he would qualify for some free tuition at the community college nearby. It seemed like such a silly thought in light of all that had happened, but it was not silly to him. Jen gave him the good news.

"The school district administrator came by last night. She said your grades are frozen where they are right now. No more tests, no more school! You will graduate with your class, and you will remain with your benefits from the A+ Program!"

Ethan was relieved.

I hugged Jen, Hannah, and Jen's mom, who were all smiles. We talked for a while. Then it was time for me to give the family some space. Ethan's girlfriend was texting their friends as tears of joy rolled down her face, and they would be arriving soon. It was their turn.

Ethan gradually came around and regained all of his functions. Doctors gave him some more tests and surgeons placed a defibrillator beneath the skin in his chest to prevent further cardiac arrests. A few days later, Ethan was diagnosed with Left Ventricular Non-Compaction Cardiomyopathy. It's a rare genetic disorder that can usually be controlled with medications and a surgically implanted defibrillator, but he might eventually need a heart transplant.

The symptoms can be as simple and subtle as tiredness. These are the kids you hear about on the TV news who drop dead on the football field. We were all thankful that Ethan had been surrounded by angels on that beautiful spring day. After nine days he was able to go home, but he had something to do first.

Ethan, Jen, Ed and their families all made a special stop on the way home. They visited his school, Eureka High School, where it happened to be Teacher Appreciation Week. They surprised the teachers and coaches gathered in the gym for an assembly honoring teachers. Ethan and his family wanted to thank the ones who were there when he collapsed, who played a crucial part in saving his life.

Someone had called the local news before they arrived and told a reporter the story. News Channel Five was there to catch the family saying thanks to their heroes.

"I didn't even know if he was going to be alive," Jen said in the TV interview. "We didn't know, when he was waking up, if he would even recognize any of us. And the first thing he said was 'Mom,' and there were just tears." She drew her hand down her cheek. "I mean, what do you say to people, who, without them, he wouldn't be here?" There was hugging and the crowd applauded the coaches and nurse. Kay Quinn, a news anchor for the station, told the story on the local news.

Jessica Patton, R.N.

In a heart attack or a full cardiac arrest there are only seconds before the body can no longer survive. The chances of survival are very slim without intervention. CPR and the availability of an AED can be critical in increasing the chances of survival.

It seemed to me, if his cardiac arrest had to happen, it had been arranged to perfection: the three coaches happened to be there at that exact time and place although it wasn't in their original plans for that day; one carried his cellphone in his pocket. The paramedics' quick response, the hospital only twelve minutes away, the low patient count in the E.R. that day—coincidence? We think not.

Jen went on to pass boards and became an R.N. Ed continues to run a successful business. Ethan earned good grades in college and helped out with the family business. And he was still in love at the time of this writing.

I am glad that it turned out this way, and Ethan and his family are eternally grateful for this village that saved his young life.

14

A Not-So-Typical Work Day

I came through the automatic sliding glass doors and entered the E.R., its rush of warmth was a stark contrast to the four degrees above zero outside, with wind gusts driving the temperature to ten below and so sharp they might have left cuts on the side of my nose. My feet carried me swiftly as I unbundled mid-gait. I nodded at the triage nurse as she cheerfully greeted us, the oncoming shifts of nurses.

Time was almost palpable in the back left portion of my head: tick-tock, tick-tock. I had arrived on time so there was no no need to stop at the first phone I saw to clock in. I could do it when I got to my floor.

I was alone in the elevator, nice because there would be no stops on the way to the top floor, the fifth, of our "new" hospital. It was about four years old then. The lobby and halls were full of soft colors, glass, tall trees, art, and couches. A water-wall about twelve feet wide gave a constant flow of cascading water from the lobby through the floor to the ground floor below.

Designed by patients, doctors and nurses, the hospital was full of high-tech equipment and little things that were supposed to be intuitive for delivering better care, such as the Medprox, which stored patients' medications in their rooms. All rooms were private. The patients liked that. But I was past my honeymoon phase, and never having worked in another adult hospital I had nothing to compare this one to. From what other nurses said, we had a lot to be thankful for.

I punched the code pad on the nurses' lounge door and it flew open, pushed from the inside by exiting staff. Instinctively I dodged it, stepping to the side.

"Oops, sorry!" exclaimed a nurse from our sister floor, Five North. I smiled and she rushed down the hall. Tick-tock, tick-tock. We're all on the same clock now. I entered and clocked in, opened my locker which had the same silly picture of myself and my family from five years before at Christmas. I rolled my eyes and again promised myself to bring a new one in.

I gathered my stethoscope and other things. I applied them all like a tool belt; pens, scissors, dry-erase marker, penlight, badge, call light monitor. I stuffed my purse into the locker, grabbed a self-made patient-organizer page, hung my coat up and exited slowly, so the door would not crack anyone in the head. Tick-tock, tick-tock.

Amy was the charge nurse. I saw that we had the normal staffing ratio of four patients each that day. We were adequately staffed. A little flutter in my belly jumped for joy. We wouldn't be asked to do the impossible today and care for more patients than we could handle on our medical-surgical floor, with no help except each other plus one aide for a total of twenty patients, most with extensive needs such as assistance to the bathroom or bedpans, assistance with eating, assistance with their unquenchable anxiety. Other hospitals actually had ratios of seven patients to one nurse. They could not possibly give good care. Tick-tock, tick-tock.

"I didn't get 5106 back. Bummer! She was so sweet!" I said, still happy about the adequate staffing. "She was president of the women's something or other, I can't remember." We referred to patients by their room numbers mainly because of the HIPAA federal privacy law and how we organized the patients in our minds. It was rare that we had a patient of such stature. People like that simply didn't seem to get sick.

"Yes, she's sweet, but we rotate her because we all need a chance to take care of her. We're sharing her," Amy said with a grin. "I heard she has a big home in Kirkwood. Renee had her the day before and really liked her, too." It was kind of rare, having a patient who wasn't confused, trying to hit the nurse, or trying to get drugs, or grouchy. People are grouchy when they don't feel well. We just smile and move on.

Most of the time we became listeners, mock-psychologists, pseudo-mothers, and cheerleaders to the sick. Sometimes it didn't work. But we always tried. It might surprise you how infrequent are the patients who are simply sick or injured, who do as their doctors instruct and make an effort to get better.

I felt light as I walked down the hall toward the rooms, because it was day two. Working twelve-hour shifts was exhausting. But the four days off every week is very seductive and addictive. When work overwhelmed me and I felt as if I couldn't go on, I remembered this. And tried to keep calm and press on.

On day two we usually had the same patients we had had the day before. There was no need to spend the first half hour looking up all of their demographic information, history, med times, doctors, chief complaints, orders, labs and tests, all while dodging call lights and finding the correct nurses to get reports from. This was the only time a nurse could learn about the patients. If all the call lights lit up, he or she would know less about the patients and would not have another chance to learn more about them until after med-passing time. Tick-tock, tick-tock.

Bed 5109 was a man who had had a stroke, moved to our floor to receive a chemo drug for his central nervous system vasculitis that only a chemo-certified nurse could give. That was me. Bed 5110 was a drug addict with pneumonia gone almost too far. She cried every time I entered the room, asking for pain medicine, and when I left she resumed her regular voice on the phone, talking while filing her nails. I knew because the double window outside her room in the hall had blinds, slightly open, in between the windows.

Bed 5119 was a very thin neglected uneducated elderly woman with 'C-Diff', the mother of all infections, causing horrible diarrhea and very hard to get rid of. Bed 5120 was a lady with asthma and according to the doctors and all the tests everything was normal. And when I assessed her she was fine, her lungs clear, with good, deep breaths, until her husband entered the room. Then there seemed to be a big show of pain and shortness of breath that wasn't there before. The symptoms disappeared when he left and the pulmonologist entered. She would probably protest being discharged that day. I hoped there was no drama. There was much drama in the medical profession.

Doctors and nurses see a lot of "fake" illness. A drug addict will come to the hospital and lie about illness to obtain narcotics. Some people come for relief from stressful home situations. The hospital might be the only peace they will have. When all the tests are run and turn up negative, these people agree and go home peacefully. A patient truly having problems will protest loudly and angrily. It can be difficult for the doctor to tell, but this might warrant further testing or recommendations. It happens much more often than people realize.

As that day went on, I had time to stop in and speak to the lady in 5106. She was about eighty years young, and her elegance, artful conversation, subtly girlish charm and southern drawl bestowed on us her wisdom. These gifts are increasingly absent in younger generations. Another nurse, Nicole, also came in while the patients' friend-visitor was there. We didn't want to intrude but she invited us. She had a kind of glow. It was rare that we had a patient Just. Be. Nice.

Are We Angels

I forgot after a few minutes that we were in her hospital room. We might have been sipping lemonade on a hot summer day on her front porch. She spoke, in her slow southern drawl, about poodles, and women, and hinted at the importance of kindness, and told us what wonderful nurses we were. She asked us about our lives and children. She told me I should join the St. Louis Writers Guild (which I did). She was delightful. Her smile was infectious, her wisdom magnetic.

Being a nurse can be incredibly stressful. The management of all of the doctors' orders, obtaining doctors' orders for things we needed or the doctor forgot, charting everything, giving meds to patients on time, doing assessments, arranging for tests and surgeries, maintaining safety for confused patients who seemed determined to hurt themselves by falling or ripping IVs or catheters out: It can be overwhelming. Then there are constant phone interruptions: call lights, calls from physical therapy and dietary, doctors, social workers, other nurses, other departments, family members. Nurses receive phone calls all day long: during patient care, during med pass, in the bathroom, and we are expected to answer. There is no voicemail. Nurses have an agenda for their days, a work schedule to keep despite the acuity of their patients, meaning how sick they are or how much personal care they need.

Nurses get tired. We get tired of computer systems or other equipment that doesn't work, constant and ever-increasing continuing education expected to be done during work hours, constant emails that don't pertain to us, systems of operation that don't work right, as well as constant change from teams put together that don't improve patient care or nursing but only make things worse. Our hospital was probably one of the best-crafted and best-staffed around. The people were great. It was like a small town. Despite the problems, I believed I was lucky to work there.

Patients don't feel well. They are going about their lives

when their body (or mind, in some cases) betrays them. They ask us for help. They usually don't have the slightest idea what is going on in their bodies and sometimes doubt what they are told. They are fearful about their prognoses. They worry about money and the very real financial burden that will result from being in the hospital. They look at themselves, their bodies and illness as a weakness and a burden and instead of being kind to themselves begin to turn against themselves in bitterness and self-loathing. Sometimes they give up. They don't follow the doctor's instructions because they lack understanding or money, and they hope for the best. Or they do everything the doctor says and still their health declines. It can be frightening being a patient.

So, here she was, this wonderful woman in bed six, having all this stress, being in the hospital, and yet going out of her way to beam hope and happiness and strength. Was that how it worked? I made a mental note (*don't let it all get to me, don't let it all get to me, help me lift someone else's spirits today*). I think I changed a little that day. I felt lighter, more at peace. I felt that maybe I could go on.

If you ever read this, dear lady in bed six, you are wonderful, and thank you. You helped me handle a burden I felt was conquering my spirit and wearing me down. I was supposed to be the giver of help, knowledge and kindness. But *you* were the little light that brightened my day.

Epilogue

So, I go on, despite feeling like a circus horse trotting around and around inside the ring. I press the feelings down, blow them off, hide them under the carpet. I look for those moments. I make a conscious effort to be positive, to see the best in people, and usually it works. I am off four days a week. I have time to help with our business and be involved with our boys. I have a steady paycheck. I work in "pajamas." I have mastered the work at the hospital, so it's comfortable and I can be on auto-pilot.

I help people. I am part of a team that improves people's lives, and brings families hope. That is in itself a miracle. I actually do work at a wonderful hospital that isn't perfect, but honestly tries to do its best for patients and staff. I've learned that self-care is not a dirty word. I have so much to be grateful for, and I am.

It's probably just me. I give one hundred and ten percent to whatever I do. I take responsibility very seriously. But is it actually ego that makes me feel the weight of the world on my shoulders, as a nurse? I feel like a failure when I think about quitting. My body aches after every shift. I no longer want to be tough. Sick, grouchy people (who obviously can't help it) can be difficult. The emotional drain is real. I don't want to lose my compassion. People deserve compassion, even the difficult ones.

I sense the curiosity and ambition of other nurses and students who remind me of my younger self. There's an almost athletic personality required for nursing that I don't have. Maybe I'm too sensitive, but that's who I am. Younger nurses are tech-y, embracing the computer work. They don't mind the constant call-lights and phone call interruptions. For me, it's overstimulation and interrupts my concentration.

It's easy to care for patients who aren't anxious or frequently incontinent or trying to hit you, or drug-seeking. But all patients need care. Despite my complaints I believe that. But because hospitals are reimbursed based on popularity surveys, nurses and other medical staff have lost control of the ability to set boundaries and limits. Rating a hospital is like rating a hotel you've stayed in. No one wants to stay in a one-star hotel, even if the rater is a drug addict angry that he didn't get his dilaudid (narcotic pain medication). But that's our system. It just is.

I'd like to say a word about money, just one word. When people are sick, when they're at their lowest, it's a kick in the groin to them to put a price tag on their bodies. I believe humans are priceless. I believe our system is arrogant and broken. Not everything needs to be for sale.

I've come a long way since I saw the nurse in the restaurant. And I love that I became a nurse, if for nothing else then to understand the physical needs of my kids. I don't want to move on, earn more degrees, or change to a different field of nursing. I think, for me, if I'm honest about it, I'm pretty much done. At least with full-time work. I don't think I'll ever fully quit. I might be exhausted and depleted, but if I focus more on setting personal boundaries, and on self-care, maybe I'll have more to offer. Maybe I'll work two days per month someday, when I have that choice.

Or maybe I'll open a little ice-cream shop. Or become a writer. It's funny, how midlife can force such a huge re-examination of one's life.

Are We Angels

I've realized over the years that one doesn't have to be a nurse to make a difference. Nursing is only one of a million ways. Anyone and everyone can make a difference, simply with kindness. I see that now. I wish that had been clearer to me all those years ago. Nurses need only that and to be fascinated with the human body to be successful.

For now, I will hold on to those moments. They do still happen. I will continue to dig deeply, seek the positive in everything and everyone, and always do my duty as a nurse no matter how I feel. If you are a patient or family of a patient, know that your caregivers are human, they are not angels, and that they went through back-breaking training and work long hours, all for you. And that we care. We cry at your losses and celebrate your successes with you. If you are at the beginning of your nursing school or career, keep going if you know it's for you. I ask only that you embrace fully the idea that when you are out there, you can do it better than I have.

Afterword

Things have changed since I started writing this book six years ago. We are now living in the pandemic of COVID-19. Many people have become sick and died. So many healthcare workers have died. At the time of this writing there are still so many questions about this virus and the treatment for it. People are tired of social distancing. People are mistrustful of those in power. They are very concerned about finances. The Dow plunged and has creeped back up but will it drop again? Airline travel has dropped 95 percent. No one knows how this will turn out.

Nurses, doctors, respiratory therapists, and many other healthcare workers are being called heroes. They are. But please consider this: We/they chose their careers, but they did not choose the hell that is the pandemic of COVID-19. The failure of the system from protecting the masses, including healthcare workers, will be remembered.

Last summer, I worked myself into a back injury. I have been on light duty and was recently told I have permanent restrictions. I am looking for more of a desk job now. My hospital has me working various jobs, mostly screening incomers at the entryways for signs of COVID-19 infection. I am fortunate to still be working.

I see the tears of family members as they drop off items for the loved ones that they cannot enter to see. I hear about the sadness of the patients battling alone, missing the touch of their families. I feel for my co-workers on the front lines, with mask pressure scars on their faces from battling this virus. They are not heroes, they are not angels. This is not some romanticized war story. This is hell.

Nurses are holding their breath for twelve or thirteen hours and doing their absolute mental, emotional, and physical best, and it's still not enough. They are your mothers, fathers, sons, daughters, sisters, brothers, friends and lovers. They are humans that happen to know some things about the body. And while they appreciate your praise, what they really need is your understanding and support. Ask them how their day was, then sit back and listen, even if it hurts. Let them know you appreciate their courage.

Because that's the thing about nurses and all healthcare workers. Once we set foot into our workplace we have no choice. Nurses and doctors don't really get to pick and choose who we care for. We care for everyone, no matter how diligent, or compliant, or complacent or destructive people are with their bodies. Much like I envision heavenly beings are for us. Are we angels? I say no, we are humans; we have limits. But then again maybe so, because we never stop trying. Because whenever there is need, we will be there. It's who we are.

About the Author

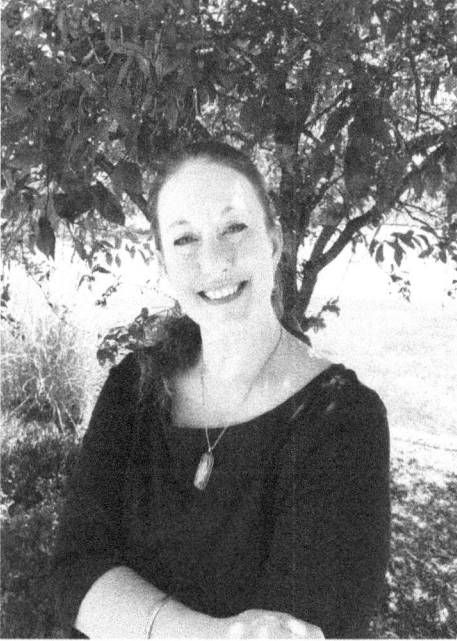

Jessica Patton is from St. Louis, MO, where she loves having three sons and running a business with her husband. She has been a nurse for 30 years. She found time to write in the earliest morning hours on her days off when it was quiet and she could share a cup of coffee with her husband and dream of becoming a writer.

www.ingramcontent.com/pod-product-compliance
Lightning Source LLC
LaVergne TN
LVHW011240080426
835509LV00005B/576